New Wives' Tales *Conversations with Parents About Today's Pediatrics*

Also by Lendon H. Smith, M.D.

THE CHILDREN'S DOCTOR
THE ENCYCLOPEDIA OF BABY AND CHILD CARE

Series Editor:
TEACHING YOUR CHILD TO LEARN
WHAT YOUR CHILD *REALLY* WANTS TO KNOW ABOUT SEX--AND *WHY*

New Wives' Tales

Conversations with Parents About Today's Pediatrics

by LENDON H. SMITH, M.D.

PRENTICE-HALL, INC.
Englewood Cliffs, New Jersey

New Wives' Tales: Conversations with Parents About Today's Pediatrics, by Lendon H. Smith, M.D.

Printed in the United States of America

Prentice-Hall International, Inc., London
Prentice-Hall of Australia, Pty. Ltd., North Sydney
Prentice-Hall of Canada, Ltd., Toronto
Prentice-Hall of India Private Ltd., New Delhi
Prentice-Hall of Japan, Inc., Tokyo

10 9 8 7

Library of Congress Cataloging in Publication Data
Smith, Lendon H.
New wives' tales.
1. Infants—Care and hygiene. I. Title.
RJ61.S663 649'.1 73–14800
ISBN 0–13–616177–4

I dedicate this book to my children —Tracy, Nancy, Eric, Duncan, and Tim— in the hopes that the precepts I have laid on them will not be too constricting. And thanks again to Peggy Moss and Nancy Elsner for editing, proofreading, and encouraging.

Contents

1

The Need for New Wives' Tales

Do you remember the picture the American Medical Association used about twenty years ago in a public relations ad promoting the good image of the doctor? It showed the dedicated doctor sitting at the bedside of a very sick child while the parents stood helplessly but confidently nearby. The lay reader was to get the impression that the doctor was available, humane, helpful, and supportive. Doctors, too, saw the ad. Young ones in training or just out in practice projected themselves into the image and hoped they would fit the conception. Older doctors thought: "The poor jerk. He doesn't know what the kid's got and he's sitting there hoping the diagnosis will come to him."

After some protest, the ad disappeared. The main criticism, I believe, was that the picture suggested that the present-day doctor was willing to make house calls.

The doctor of that bygone era sat at the bedside, showed his love for humanity, and waited for the crisis. His concerned visage might have masked his feelings of inadequacy, but it was interpreted by patient and family to be an expression of hope. His wisdom and strength were sometimes sufficient to encourage the patient to survive. His presence in the sickroom was frequently associated with the patient's improvement, so he was occasionally given credit for the cure. This implied but fortuitous causal relationship was rewarding to the doctor, psychologically as well as financially, so he continued to respond to the sick call.

As time passed and science improved technology, certain methods of treatment were found to improve the patient's chance of cure, so they were continued and other less reliable therapeutics were abandoned (bloodletting, enemas to eliminate poisons, cauterizing wounds, water immersion for witchcraft, trephining for epilepsy).

In the last thirty years, since sulfa and penicillin were discovered, the medical axiom has been for a specific treatment for each specific disease or condition. Since the success of therapy hinged on the accuracy of the diagnosis, all medical school training was directed to instilling in the doctor the information necessary to achieve an exact diagnosis. Don't just relieve the symptoms (for example, by prescribing aspirin for headache, purge for constipation), find out *why* the symptoms are present. A certain constellation of symptoms and signs suggests a number of diseases. Further history, questions, the examination, laboratory tests, and X-ray examination *should* lead to one disease. Then, if one forgets which medicine or what dose is called for, a medical book with a good index will practically write out the prescription or the type of surgery required.

The doctor has a million facts stored away in his memory, retrievable, we all hope, at the appropriate time. He invested time, money, and anxiety in learning them so he would be able to help his patients. Anyone who would subject himself to all this education must use it; if it doesn't work, then all these labors have been in vain.

One night in the emergency room of a large hospital a drunk was brought in by the police. He seemed to be in some discomfort, so he needed to be checked out before they threw him in the drunk tank. The intern on duty could find nothing wrong, and the semicomatose patient was unable to give any sort of information except to groan and clutch his abdomen.

Drunks can be a diagnostic challenge, as they may have diabetes, pancreatitis, coronary occlusion, or a broken bone. Blood tests were normal, so the fledgling doctor felt he'd better get an X ray in order to rule out intestinal obstruction. The film revealed the distinct outline of a Coca-Cola bottle securely sequestered in his rectum.

This was a new syndrome to the doctor, who had learned everything they laid on him in medical school. The Intern's Manual had no reference to this under "bottle," "cola syrup," or "rectum." Time was running out, as the anesthetic benefits of the alcohol were disappearing. He was forced to call the resident on duty, the next man up in the hierarchy of emergency care—a nervous, tense, restless man who occasionally made a mere emergency a catastrophe. The resident's response to the problem of "pelvic foreign object" was to dash up to the obstetrical department to borrow the forceps; his plan was to deliver the bottle while the patient was still under twilight sleep!

This was an old hospital and needed overhauling. The excited resident opened the elevator door and stepped in to find the elevator was missing. He fell about six feet to the greasy bottom of the shaft, breaking both wrists. The orthopedic surgeon casted his arms; meanwhile the hospital engineer drilled a hole into the bottom of the bottle and extracted the foreign body. For some months after this the resident kept the X ray above his mantle like a trophy to remind himself of the most fascinating case he had attended.

Doctors delight in the unusual, the complicated—but solvable—mysteries of the human body. Thirty years ago I read the case history of a banker who had a severe, constant, unignorable crotch itch. The dermatologist reporting the case was ecstatic because (1) it was unusual and (2) he solved it. The doctor took some pictures of the red, excoriated area (some psychiatrists think dermatologists are really "respectable" voyeurs), searched for anything moving, took scrapings for fungus, cultures for bacteria, asked about changes of soap or new material in the underwear. Nothing. The mystery deepened. A psychological problem was considered, but the man denied any business or domestic disorder. The banker was even asked to make a list of his daily activities.

It was practically an emergency situation. Few people want to leave money in a bank where one of the officers has a problem that suggests an unsavory private life.

The banker's (and the dermatologist's) reputation was saved by the discovery of the cause. This busy executive was having his daily elimination after breakfast, reading the *Wall Street Journal* while simultaneously shaving with one of the new electric razors. At that time these clippers had no hair catchers, and the spray of shorn stubble was being funneled by the newspaper into the above-mentioned area.

The patient was unable to make the connection between the symptom and the cause. The doctor knew there was a connection and persevered until he reached the solution: The doctor is happiest when allowed to make the diagnosis.

Most doctors nowadays are goal oriented; they set up an end and then strive to attain it. (Some would say this tendency is the result of over toilet training.) It has been shown that this desire to achieve may be inborn but is usually fostered by parents who "want the best for my son." High standards of performance may have been set in the home and then become a part of the personality structure. Essentially the doctor plays this game with himself all his life. Find a problem, solve it. The doctor wants to be the scientific detective and solve the riddle of the illness.

If he cannot diagnose the case before him, or is not allowed to, he is unable to justify his degree. He must be successful or he becomes frustrated. By the diploma on his wall he has declared to his patients and his colleagues (and the world) that he is a physician or surgeon. If the diagnosis does not come bubbling up to his conscious level after the data have been fed into his brain, he feels guilty.

Dermatologists are frequently derogated by their professional peers because they deal so often with non-life-threatening conditions. Again, the most destructive blow to their ego comes from the many patients who appear with the diagnosis already established. The first and most important step to the cure has already been usurped by the patient.

"Doc, I've got this wart, see."

"Yes, you have a verrucous excrescence."

"Okay, can you do something about my acne?" or "What do you have for poison oak?" It all seems to have deteriorated to the level of the supermarket.

No wonder dermatologists (and all the rest of us) get excited about the diagnostic challenge: the patient who comes "clean" to the office with an occult problem. But if you march in with a page from the *Reader's Digest* listing all the symptoms of infectious mononucleosis and state that your fifteen-year-old has it, the doctor may feel compelled to sabotage your diagnosis by discovering some social disease. How much better for all to play the game by the house rules. "He has had a sore throat, fever, swollen neck glands, and a headache for the past ten days. We gave him penicillin for a few days, but he got worse. We are so worried. Would you help us?" The doctor knows that penicillin always works on a strep throat so he feels for and finds an enlarged spleen. He suspects mononucleosis, does a blood test, and confirms his suspicions. Everybody wins. The patient is really the winner in the doctor's office if he is aware of the doctor's strong need to "crack the case."

New Wives' Tale: The doctor* needs *to help you.

Old Wives' Tale: "The doctor wants to help you."

Rules to follow if you or your child has a new condition or disease or fever or itch or sudden stomach ache:

1. Ask for the doctor's help; appeal to the Albert Schweitzer humanitarian sometimes latent under the scientist.

2. Never state the diagnosis; that is his job and the main reason he stays in business.

3. Try to list the problems separately and in their order of appearance. "He was perfectly well until five

days ago, when . . . ." The doctor recognizes a disease by the course it usually takes.

4. Try to let the doctor decide if the patient needs to be examined. If you *insist* on a house call, he may come, but will act like a noncompliant, glumpy, three-year-old who feels put down by his rigid mother. The doctor must feel *he* is making the decision.

Of course, it helps if a doctor is somewhat overcontrolled, rigid, self-sacrificing, and somewhat compulsive to do well academically, but these very attributes may prevent him from being sympathetic toward the patient whose life style is a little "loose." Ill-concealed contempt may negate any therapy dependent on a good working relationship. The doctor feels, "I was able to overcome obstacles; you can also." He frequently cannot help patients whose problems seem to stem from self-indulgence.

"My twelve-year-old daughter is fat. I'd like to do something now. My whole adolescence was miserable because I was a fat slob and nobody did anything for me. Is it her glands? She eats very little but has gained fifteen pounds this past year."

I am flattered that I have been asked to help. I know it is going to be tough to break a twelve-year habit of taking more calories than are burned up, but I'm willing to try. The girl has grown two to three inches a year, her skin is warm and moist, and her thyroid test is normal. She is not anemic, school is okay, she has friends, and the domestic scene has the average ups and downs. She is just fat; she has learned to disregard some message in her hypothalamus that she has eaten enough.

"Okay," I say, "here is a sensible 1,500-calorie diet.

It has the right proportion of carbohydrate, protein, and fat. You must exercise at least an hour a day." I address the girl and hope some hypnotic influence will motivate her to follow my instructions. "Do you want to lose weight?"

"Oh, yes," she intones mechanically, glancing at her mother. I ignore this premonition of failure.

"Let's set our goals realistically. If you can keep your weight gain to six to ten pounds a year, you will grow into your weight and in a couple of years your hormones will move your fat deposits around to the appropriate areas. Okay? Come back in a month and we'll see what happens."

Mother and daughter return in a month. Weight gain: three pounds. "We really tried. How about those water pills? Maybe it's water she can't flush out."

"Okay, okay. Here's a prescription. See you in a month."

It is no surprise that the patient fails to return. A phone call about a rash a few months later reminds me: "How's the weight problem?" I ask, cringing.

"Oh, that. We joined Weight Watchers and we're both losing three to four pounds a month. Thanks anyway." I simply call in an expensive ointment for the rash.

A doctor likes to win. When he outlines a program and the patient does not follow it, it is difficult for him to accept the responsibility for the therapeutic failure. The patient is blamed. He seeks help elsewhere—which is what the doctor wanted in the first place. Don't allow the failure to return.

Office visit: "We can't do anything with this child. He's five years old and is disobedient and mean. He refuses to do anything we ask. He won't eat or go to bed. He calls us names. Discipline just makes him want to get revenge. He was thrown out of kindergarten because he fights, breaks chalk, and gooses the girls. I can't stand him. My husband thinks he is just being a boy and laughs at his antics, but then he's gone all day and only sees him a couple of hours in the evening. I cry myself to sleep because I know I'm a lousy mother; my mother-in-law tells me so."

In the time it takes for the mother to relate the above story, the doctor has made a diagnosis of poor impulse control in a child who has not been disciplined properly. The stethoscope has been jerked from his ears, he has been kicked in the groin, and he could not get the boy's underwear off for the hernia check. From his own childhood and what he learned in school, the doctor *knows* that the child has not been disciplined enough. His answer to the parents is, "He's got to learn to control his impulses and you've got to teach him."

Lack of self-control is not part of a doctor's mental makeup; it is foreign to him, like trying to understand color blindness without having had the experience. The fact that the parents have tried rigid control and firm, even punitive, discipline does not impress the doctor. He was told in medical school by the psychiatric department that behavior problems are environmentally produced, and the environment (that is, the parents) must change. His own children responded to discipline; others can also. He finds no neurological disorder that could explain it; therefore poor parenting must be responsible. The doctor doesn't know that some chemical-neurological defect in the inhibitory control network of the brain is responsible. He cannot see it or test for it, so he cannot diagnose it by the methods he learned in school. Because the condition is not stored in his memory as a medically treatable condition, he can only respond with, "See a psychiatrist" or "He'll outgrow it."

Another frustrating problem: "Our child seems slow. He didn't sit until he was a year old and walked at twenty months. Speech now at age three years is an unintelligible word salad. We have been told to stimulate him with stories, games, and a thing called patterning and he will come out of it."

The doctor notes that the parents carefully avoid the use of the charged word, "retardation" so *he* circumvents it also. He is interested in the case until he rules out correctable problems: hydrocephalus, PKU, low thyroid, lead poisoning, anemia, low-protein diet, deprivation. These are "fun" things to handle because the doctor can use his stored information to diagnose and treat them. But the vast majority of retardates have been hurt by genetic or intrauterine influences not correctable by present techniques. The diagnosis may be clear-cut, but the doctor cannot move to the next step, the successful treatment. What is the point of naming the illness if there is no solution?

"Well, he's retarded," he responds a little angrily. The parents get the message: Don't come back here; you make the doctor uncomfortable.

These few examples point up the chief gap in this otherwise near perfect picture of the doctor: his inability to accept the fact that he cannot cure everything and that sympathetic understanding or willingness to share the burden of unfortunate conditions is really part of his job. He needs to remember the old slogan, "Relieve guilt and suffering." The doctor should not become angry at the diabetic for not producing enough insulin nor at the obese patient for absorbing too many calories. Sympathy and understanding are important methods of treatment also. Many conditions can only be controlled; at least the burden can be shared.

Although medical school teaching is improving in encouraging young doctors to be more accepting of life styles, many of us in practice are still driving patients out of our offices. The mutually supportive lay groups such as Alcoholics Anonymous, National Association for Mentally Retarded, Cystic Fibrosis Association, Suicide Prevention Centers, Epilepsy League, Weight Watchers, TOPS, La Leche League, and many others all attest to the dissatisfaction of large groups of people with the performance of doctors in dealing with various specific conditions. (There is no pneumonia or strep throat fund because the doctors can deal with these effectively.)

Guilt, anger, and frustration, then, motivate the parents to seek help elsewhere, usually not from an M.D.'s office. Are sympathy and understanding incompatible with the scientific approach?

New Wives' Tale: Doctors should at least make you feel better.

"Doctors can cure anything nowadays."

Rules to follow if you or your child has a chronic condition already diagnosed (thumb-sucking, bed-wetting, hyperactivity, dyslexia, truancy, obesity, epilepsy, mental retardation, cystic fibrosis, allergy, diabetes, rheumatic fever, depression, kidney failure, alcoholism, hemophilia, cancer, leukemia):

1. Find out by word, action, facial expression if your doctor is able and willing to treat, maintain, control, support, encourage, empathize with you.

2. Contact the local, state, or national organization involved with the condition. Your local medical society can help: a nearby medical school may be the nucleus of research in the problem. These groups are able to provide names of doctors who are interested or willing or able to provide the help, expertise, hope, or support that you need.

Part of the problem, I think, is that doctors often feel impatient with parents who haven't kept up with the times. Retardation, diabetes, even venereal disease are all out in the open, widely discussed, so we doctors assume that our patients are at least familiar with them. It is devastating, of course, to have a doctor suggest a disease or syndrome you never even suspected, but imagine the doctor's position! He is all ready to write out the prescription, and suddenly realizes he's left the parent way behind and has to pause to fill her in on what's been happening in medicine these past thirty years. We like to be able to provide the fruits of our medical experience; we don't want to have to repeat the whole course each time we talk to a new mother.

In short, medicine has changed and doctors have changed, but the patients haven't. A broken leg hurts just as much as it did back in frontier days. We doctors assume, however, that the patient should be reassured that his leg will be set in a plaster cast and not with splints of kindling. We assume that our patients know what's new in medicine and so their worries should be over. But it just isn't so.

In my two previous books, *The Children's Doctor* and *The Encyclopedia of Baby and Child Care,* I tried to give worried parents the background and "inside" information that their own doctor has but usually hasn't the time to explain in detail. But it seems that the image of that old-time Doc who stayed by the bedside is still firmly entrenched in the minds of mothers across the land. He may have an answering service and a nurse, but deep in your heart you still believe that he's the same old Doc. A pundit once said that most Englishmen believe that if you woke a Frenchman in the middle of the night, he'd speak English. A lot of parents, I think, believe that if they call at the right moment, they'll reach the "real" Doc, the same kindly, patient man who sat by their bedside and let them play with his vest-pocket watch when they were children.

"Old Wives' Tales" is the best name for this kind of deeply held belief. In your waking moments it's penicillin, DPT (diphtheria-pertussis-tetanus shot) boosters, and IQ tests, but wake up in the middle of the night, and bang!—it's mud for a bee sting. In times of fear, surprise, or emergency, we all revert to our most basic thoughts. The only difference is that for a doctor, his intern days flash before his eyes. For a parent, it's what grandmother said you ought to do. Again and again I find that parents still have a secret shelf of "home remedies" deep in their minds, and until I tell them otherwise, they'll stick to those Old Wives' Tales, regardless.

Hence this book. I want to go over those time-honored, but time-wasting root assumptions all of us have, and try to bring them up to date. It's much easier to remember "A stitch in time saves nine" than "Procrastination is counterproductive in 85 percent of students at the grade school level." So if I can boil down what I've learned and observed into some pithy *New* Wives' Tales, you will be more likely to recall them when you need them most. When you call the doctor, you'll both be speaking the same language—well, not exactly the same lingo, but the generation gap will be bridged. He'll say it in medical terms, and you'll suddenly realize he's reciting a New Wives' Tale, and you can smile knowingly and let him proceed—without that lingering doubt that grandmother said it should be done *this* way.

For example:

"When you are sick, call the doctor."

"My child had a temperature of 103° last night, and your answering service said you were off call and I would have to talk to your partner. He doesn't know my child and I'm used to talking to you. When I first came to you I thought you'd be available when I needed you."

"Well, I'm sorry, but I do need some time off to stare into space and be some sort of husband and father. Did my partner help you?"

"He said to give aspirin and a bath and call back if it didn't work."

"That sounds about like what I would have had you do. Did it help?"

"Yes, he was better in a couple of hours, but I felt so nervous, lonely, and almost abandoned. Shouldn't he have been seen last night? What if it had been pneumonia or polio or some dread disease? How would I know?"

"I can understand your concern. A fever in the child next door is just a fever, but when it's your own child, it frequently looks like an emergency. What we doctors are trying to do is get people to realize that fevers and colds and stomach aches and diarrhea are a natural part of a child's growth. He must get these virus diseases so his body can exercise its immune system. About 85 percent of the infections he gets are due to viruses; they are untreatable and considered innocuous. An average child gets six to eight respiratory infections a year. All we can do is suggest remedies that provide comfort —aspirin, decongestants, cough syrups. We believe parents should automatically supply sickness care; then, if these home measures don't work, the doctor should be consulted. If your child is hungry, you feed him. By the same token, if he's sick, you nurse him."

"How do I know when I should stop being a nurse and call in the doctor?"

"You should have some guidebook about childhood sickness that will tell you what to do for the common problems and indicate when you need some professional medical skills. All bookstores have a variety of these encyclopedias, almanacs, health guides, and the like. They all say about the same thing."

"Are you telling me that I call too much?"

"Not exactly. But why didn't you automatically give aspirin and a hot bath when the fever appeared?"

(I am saying that, in general, pediatricians, and other doctors, get too many calls about sickness which should be handled some other way. Most of us get twenty to fifty phone calls a day. This cuts into the time we should be spending on the office patients or illnesses that directly involve our specific skills. We figure at least half of the calls we get need not be answered by a doctor. A nurse could answer them, but why doesn't the lay person know the answer?)

"I guess I needed you to tell me it was okay to give the aspirin. I read somewhere the patient is supposed to have faith in the doctor. I have faith in you because you reassure me and I feel you know me and my worries and fears."

"Thank you. We like to feel needed and useful, but there should be a better balance between what *you* do and what *we* do."

There is a point beyond which doctoring should not go. Some crippled people need all the help they can get; however, most people of normal and above average IQ can often figure out what to do. If the doctor does it all, then the child almost becomes *his* baby. Let him help, encourage, back up your decisions, but you do the work. Recently in our town a doctor who was terribly conscientious wanted his new mothers to call him about anything, night or day, to get him involved in problem solving. If the baby sneezed twice, he would suggest a house call to ward off pneumonia. Parents were afraid to try out their own methods and became dependent on him. The doctor became overworked and depressed when he could not solve everything for everybody. Doctors are programmed to respond to certain symptoms that require medical intervention, but most of the daily nitty-gritties the mother must solve at the moment they occur. Baby cries; feed. Baby is wet; change. This is the beginning of parental responsibility. The doctor should be a friend and counselor, not a lover or third parent.

If you struggle through a few of the pains, drippy noses, and fevers of your children, you will begin to feel that you are in charge. You will become a better parent and will be able to cope with the more important personality growth.

"So when he is sick, I should just treat the symptoms without knowing what disease he has?"

"Something like that. When he's dirty, you bathe him. When he's tired, you put him to bed. I think what bothers most people is not having a *name* for the illness;

it is easier to deal with something if it is labeled. We often don't know what disease the child has in the first few hours or day. The symptoms are frequently nonspecific, so nonspecific methods are used until it can be determined which way the disease is going."

"Shouldn't I know right away if he has the flu or pneumonia?"

"It's worthwhile because we can treat pneumonia. Usually, but not always, home measures will temporarily control flu and other virus infections, and the chances are about nine to one against something more serious or bacterial. But even some bacterial infections don't have to be treated immediately. Evidence indicates that allowing a person to fight a bacterial infection for a few hours or a day or two teaches the body a few lessons in immunity development which will come in handy at the next attack."

New Wives' Tale: If home measures make the victim more comfortable, a few hours or a day or so can be permitted to elapse before the doctor needs to be summoned.

"I think I like what you're saying but it does put a burden of responsibility on me to cry 'Help!' at the proper time. My neighbor's doctor insists that she come to his office with every fever. He does an exam, blood count, urinalysis, X-ray, 'just to be sure.' The child has had six $20 colds in the last nine months. Why does he do all that?"

"He may be insecure about his diagnostic ability. Maybe he missed a diagnosis and he's running scared. Your neighbor may be indicating overconcern, so he feels he must go through all this to reassure her."

Doctors *are* human beings and are subject to error.

Although breakthroughs on viruses, cancer, and psychoses are imminent, we are still confronted with many patients who refuse to get well or get sicker when we treat them; or who develop allergies to the medicine or develop resistant germs or fungus diseases because of the treatment. Sometimes patients, for a variety of reasons, may not give the doctor all the facts. We can diagnose 75 percent of diseases by history alone. The exam, lab work, and X rays will confirm the diagnosis and get the accuracy rate up to 95 percent. Sometimes patients will tell us there is a temperature of 102° when they did not take it but the child seemed warm. (One reported a 102.6° temperature, but we eventually traced it to a previous fever; she had not shaken down the thermometer.)

When we suspect an allergy we have learned to ask a global question such as; "Does he fool with his nose?" If we ask, "Does he *pick* his nose?" the parent might answer, "No," because he only rubs it. We need to know if his nose itches. Diagnostic errors sometimes occur because we don't ask the right question.

"Sometimes—I hate to admit it—the doctor may not read parental concern properly at 10:00 P.M. He may feel the rash or the stool count could have waited until the next day's office hours and hence he conveys some irritation over the phone. He may know enough about learning theory that he will not reward the parent with cheerfulness; a mother might discover that a 10:00 P.M. phone call gets the doctor faster without being blocked by a cold receptionist."

"Okay, okay, I'll call during office hours. Thanks for the lecture. I've got to run. My boy is sick and I must go take care of him."

When you go to see a doctor, you must fit yourself

into his scheme of things. First, ask for his help; don't assume he will give it to you. A simple declarative sentence will do: "Please, I need your help." Second, don't state the diagnosis; this is his job, and the real reason he has studied so hard. If you think your child is anemic, don't ask for a blood count. Tell the doctor the symptoms. "My child looks pale and washed out. He eats poorly, drags around, whines, and wants to go to bed." If this doesn't suggest the child needs a blood count, or at least some iron, try, "My in-laws are on my back to find out what's wrong."

New Wives' Tale: When all else fails, treat the doctor as a sane, intelligent human being who may be saddled with a few old wives' tales himself.

2

The New Baby

(Well, today I had a baby. I'm still in one piece although I thought for a while there I was going to separate. Why do I ache all over? I feel as if someone had been beating me. The baby—Mark is his name—cried right away and my obstetrician said he was perfect. He asked for the name of a pediatrician to call in. How should I know? Does it mean the baby is not *all right? Why do we need a specialist if he is okay? We can hardly pay the bills now. Mother will help, and I have all those books so I can figure out what to do. But I'm so tired. I won't be able to read, let alone turn the pages. Nosy Mabel next door will surely know what to do.)*

New Wives' Tale: Mabel may, but the fun is in learning.

"Oh dear, there are so many things I should know and I don't. Where do I start? I feel so stupid."

"Now, now, little mother, just relax." (Beware of the doctor who calls you this. He is jockeying for position and is ranking you.) "He will let you know if he needs you. *You do what you have to do.* You will soon learn his language, and your responses will be natural and automatic."

(Here comes the nurse with Mark now. Why does he look so squashed up? He looks like Winston Churchill.) "Is that my baby?" (His wrist tag has my name on it, so I guess he is. He's funny looking but I love him. Wait until I get you home so I can cuddle you and take care of you. You're all wrapped up—I can't get next to you.)

(I'm a mother. Wow! I'm going to do it right. Not the way my mother did. Unfair, unorganized, inconsistent, indifferent. She always seemed to get mad about the wrong things. She was really okay, but it could have been better.)

Old Wives' Tale: "If a pregnant woman eats strawberries, her baby will be born with strawberry-red spots on his skin."

"I ate some strawberries a couple of months ago, and now my new baby has a red area on his wrist. I know it's nonsense, but I need you to tell me I didn't do anything wrong."

"Okay, you did nothing wrong. Even thinking evil thoughts or having bad dreams will not mark the baby. Smoking, eating a low-protein diet, taking certain drugs, and having some nasty diseases like diabetes, hypertension, severe anemia, and toxemia may predispose to inadequate fetal nutrition. Please relax and enjoy him. If you are having fun, he will get the message that he is wanted."

"You're telling me more than I need to know."

"We're trying to get people to stop worrying about the wrong things."

New Wives' Tale: If a baby has a strawberry mark, he may be the lost Prince of Silesia.

"A baby born with bumps on his head is a child of the devil. The bumps are his horns."

(What is this knob on one side of his head? A tumor? Was he dropped? It seems squishy.) "The doctor says the baby has a cephalohematoma; I made him spell it for me. Grandmother says it's a devil's horn. Should I laugh or cry?"

"It should be no problem. (A soft swelling halfway between the ear and the top of the head is a cephalohematoma, a collection of blood on the skull bone.) It heals all by itself. It is the result of an injury during birth, usually when the baby's head impinges on the mother's pelvic bone. A membrane over the bone, the periosteum, is separated from the bone by a blood clot. This swelling is squishy. The periosteum deposits calcium into this clot and so it becomes bone hard in a couple of weeks. This might suggest horns to the superstitious, but eventually it is reabsorbed and melts into the head."

New Wives' Tale: A baby with bumps on his head may have a headache, but his brain inside is okay.

"There's a scale on his head. I suppose he's got that what do they call it?—crib crust or cradle crap or cap. It's right on his soft spot. I'd better not touch it—his brain is right there. Oh dear, I can see his pulse beating. Is that okay?"

"Yes. The fontanel at the top of the head is not calcified at birth, in order to allow for molding of the skull bone during birth and to allow for growth of the brain. The skin and membranes over the brain in that area are as tough as thick canvas and can be safely fondled, washed, brushed. Being flexible, they reflect the pulse of the blood pumping into the arteries in the brain."

"If a navel looks odd, it is the obstetrician's fault."

"My baby is two months old and his belly button keeps bulging out every time he cries or strains. Did the obstetrician tie off the cord properly?"

"He probably didn't. He is so busy at that moment of truth, he usually delegates the job to the O.R. nurse."

"You mean a nurse did it?"

"He clamps it, cuts it, hands the baby to the nurse, and then awaits the passage of the placenta. The nurse puts a special clip or cloth tie on the stump just a quarter- or half-inch away from the skin edge. This keeps the vessels from leaking blood before the stump dries up."

"What keeps the intestines from falling out?"

"The opening through which the cord blood vessels pass is surrounded by elastic tissue which contracts and narrows this opening in most babies—but not yours, obviously. In some children it takes years for this opening to close. Until then you must get used to the bulge—hernia really."

"Do I put a fifty cent piece on it?"

"Save your money. When you come in next, I'll tape it for you so you won't have to look at it. Taping may make it disappear a little faster. Remember the pictures in *National Geographic* of the native families? The parents have nice, small, flat navels, but many of the children have umbilical hernias. I have to assume that these bulges disappear without surgery. So take heart."

New Wives' Tale: An umbilical hernia is a genetic defect and not an obstetrical error.

"Wait until the umbilical cord is completely healed before giving a baby a bath."

"When can I bathe my baby? The cord remnant is still on."

"You could have bathed him yesterday. Really, it's all right, but actually they don't get that dirty. Just a little soap is to be used—just enough to make the skin slippery. The rinsing with warm water may be more effective in cleansing the skin."

"Will water run into him through the navel?"

"No, it's all sealed off. The blood-encrusted navel stump is a good place for germs to grow; cleaning washes off these germs. Don't use alcohol (too drying) or baby lotions (may cause rash); use a dab of some antibiotic ointment. This will kill a few bacteria and keep the area soft and pliable. If the stump gets hard and dry, it often cracks and bleeds."

"What kind of soap, oil, and ointment should I use?"

"Really, the less the better."

Most soaps are alkaline and irritate the skin. An acid soap without hexachlorophene is the best because it cleans without alkalizing. Baby oils are perfumed and may cause rashes. Mineral oil and/or lanolin is safe. Heavy zinc ointments are safe to apply on the skin to protect it from urine or stool maceration. Don't use cotton-tipped applicators to remove wax from ears or crust from nose; the material is usually pushed farther into the orifice.

New Wives' Tale: If he has a disagreeable odor, bathe him.

"You can spoil a baby by picking him up every time he cries."

Possibly, but it's the quality and timing that make the difference. In the first three months the baby should be picked up, cuddled, loved, and told over and over again that he is wanted and someone cares. Fifteen or twenty minutes of loud bellowing compel the normally aware parent to feed, change, burp, soothe, rock—do something. After three months or so the baby should begin to realize that help for his needs is on the way; he becomes able to suppress his demands for immediate gratification if he can see or hear or feel his mother nearby. He knows she will do something to make him comfortable very soon. She also learns how quickly she must get to him to feed or change before he flies into an irreversible rage. This holding action of delaying impulse gratification can be extended over longer periods of time as long as he eventually gets satisfied. He learns that to be socially acceptable he must control his impulses. The adult counterpart is the ability to saddle oneself with a twenty-year mortgage before achieving home ownership.

A doctor once said, "Don't pick up or soothe a baby when he is crying or he will be encouraged to cry for attention." This seems antihuman, but he makes a point: people learn certain behavior more quickly if they are rewarded by love or attention. Mothers realize that the helpless, hungry, wet baby must be satisfied immediately; in the first few weeks his demands are emergencies. Once he is programmed to know that he will get his reward, he can utilize inhibitory control. But his nervous system has not developed the various selective inhibitory systems that allow *him* to allow *his mother* to talk him out of reacting explosively to his churning stomach or his burning buttocks. The mother can usually do this at about three or four months of age, but it is a gradual process. Some children never seem to acquire this trait; they are considered immature, or they may have minimal cerebral dysfunction, a neurological rather than a psychiatric disorder.

New Wives' Tale: You can spoil a **child** ***or an*** **adult** ***by picking him up every time he cries.***

"Bright lights will damage a baby's eyes."

"My husband wants to take some flash pictures of the baby and I won't let him. Doesn't that sudden bright light hurt his eyes?"

"Not really. He will blink and jerk his head away, but the light itself will not cause any damage. It is probably more comfortable to him than the photoflood lights that stay on for a longer time."

"Then any light is okay?"

"Artificial light is fine, but if direct sunlight is allowed to focus on the retina, a permanent blind spot will form. Even using colored glass will not protect the eye when the viewer is watching, for example, the sun's eclipse. Only indirect viewing is safe."

New Wives' Tale: Take pictures of the baby; he'll never be that cute again.

"A baby gets cross-eyed if objects are placed too close to his face."

"My sister made a mobile for the baby and thinks it should hang directly over the crib so he can entertain himself when he is not eating or sleeping. Won't he get cross-eyed?"

"He may, but not from that. We all converge our eyes when we look at close-up objects, but they don't get stuck that way unless something is wrong with the nerves or the muscles that have to do with eyeball movement. Sometimes one eye is nearsighted and one is farsighted, so binocular vision is impossible and one eye will turn to avoid a confusing double image. Sometimes there is a family trait."

"No one here has trouble."

"Do his eyes work together?"

"Yes, but they seem a little crossed already."

"Sometimes that is because some extra skin covers the inner corner of the eyes making them appear turned in. There are some simple tests we can do to see if you need an ophthalmologist."

New Wives' Tale: Eyes cross if they are going to cross.

"Colic is due to cold feet and hands."

"My baby cries and fusses all the time. He spits up some, seems full of gas, and has sloppy stools. When he is really bad in the evening, his hands and feet are like ice. My mother says if I'd put booties and mittens on him he would be calm and happy. Is this crazy?"

"Maybe, but I won't knock it. A pediatrician reported in a medical journal that he had mothers put booties on babies that were colicky and more than half reported the babies were more comfortable. I have believed that the cold extremities were due to the diversion of the circulation to the overly active gut so there wasn't enough blood to keep the hands and feet warm. It would be analogous to the cold, clammy hands you get when you have intestinal flu."

"You think the baby has the flu?"

"No. He is probably an overreactor. He may grow up to be sensitive or even hyperactive. I read of a study done on some migraine sufferers. Their hands were icy when the blood was pounding through the painfully dilated vessels in their heads. The experimenter got them to think 'warm hands.' A number of the victims could abort the headaches when they talked themselves into warm hands. Maybe some colic is an abdominal migraine."

"Theories. Give me something practical for now."

"Try soy bean milk, make the nipple holes bigger, maintain a calm environment, and I'll call in some sedative to quiet his awareness of the messages he gets from his crampy intestines. If he gets cramps, the skin is cool to touch just as adults turn pale when they have cramps. Try the booties also. Keep the room a comfortable 65° to 70° and dress him in clothes that would be of suitable weight for you."

New Wives' Tale: There are about twenty causes of colic. Cold hands and feet may be one cause, but usually they are but a sign that colic is present.

"If a baby smothers, the parents must have done something wrong."

"The three-month-old baby next door died suddenly in the middle of the night. This just confirms what I've suspected; the parents are neglectful in some way. Surely they would have noticed something the day before and at least would have called the doctor. Was it an old sagging mattress that caused it? I didn't think these things happened any more."

"Crib death is actually the most common cause of death in the two- to ten-month-old age group. We are really helpless when we are summoned in the morning to pronounce a baby dead and know that he had been lively, smiling, and eating well the day before. Our stupid, 'It's one of those things,' is less than consoling to the distraught, guilt-laden parents. They often feel that if they had just gone in and checked the baby one more time before they retired, they might have averted the tragedy."

"What *did* they do wrong?"

"They didn't do anything wrong. The brightest minds in the pediatric field have not found the cause. But parental neglect has not been a factor. We know what other things are *not* responsible: low gamma globulin, pneumonia, smothering, cerebral hemorrhage, milk allergy, heart failure. It is possible that a sudden, overwhelming, virus infection might trigger what appears to be a death by asphyxia. Our biggest problem is to keep the parents from disintegrating when this unheralded death hits them. Because we are so unsure of the cause, it makes it difficult for us to be reassuring. Because the death is sudden, the coroner and the police are frequently brought in, which suggests some criminal action."

New Wives' Tale: Sudden infant death must be blamed on the medical profession's inability to solve the mystery.

"Babies have a fever when they are teething."

"My year-old baby has had a fever for a week. I know it's from teething, but how long is it safe to give aspirin?"

"Whoops. A fever shouldn't last more than 72 hours without investigation. You don't have my book."

"He's just cut all his four molars. Doesn't that cause a fever?"

"I think babies are more prone to the invasion of viruses when teeth erupt. Maybe the hole in the gum allows the virus to get into the system. But the teeth pushing through don't cause the fever."

"He's got a runny nose and won't take his bottle. Surely that is teeth."

"Upper teeth eruption cause the nose to run, and lower teeth eruption create a cough, probably due to local blood vessel congestion. Bottle refusal usually means an ear infection; the vacuum created by the sucking pulls on the tender eardrums. By the way, what is the color of the mucus from his nose?"

"Chartreuse."

"That's a bacterial infection. He needs an antibiotic. Can you bring him down?"

New Wives' Tale: Babies may have sore gums when they are teething, but most fevers are due to viruses.

"Clip the tongue-tie to prevent stuttering later on."

"My mother says the baby has a tongue-tie and if it's not fixed, he may stutter when he is three years old. Did you notice it when you examined him in the hospital?"

"Why . . . ah . . . yes, but I didn't mention it because I didn't think people believed that anymore. Now I know what your mother thinks; what do *you* think?"

"I don't know. That's why I'm calling. You're the expert. Shall I call a speech therapist?"

"It is true that many three-year-olds stutter or stammer and a few of these have a short frenum holding the tongue down, but there is no evidence that there is any connection unless the parents *believe* there is a relationship. Parents who overreact to the normal stammering of the three-year-old who says, 'I . . . I . . . I . . . go . . . go . . . go . . .' will often fix the child in this pattern."

"Will you clip it?"

"Okay. I'll be glad to, but I'll just be perpetuating the myth. I can nick that membrane to make the tongue more mobile, if you promise not to freak out when he stammers in a few years."

"I promise."

"I hate to tell you this, but there are rare reports of alarming bleeding after this clipping."

"Thanks."

New Wives' Tale: A tongue-tie bothers only those who have to look at it.

"Babies must have stiff shoes when they first walk or they will become flat-footed."

"My baby is a year old and has just begun to stand up holding on to the furniture. My mother wants to get him some shoes. I'd just as soon let him go barefoot, but as long as she is going to pay for them I guess I'll let her do it. What kind are best?"

"If she wants to do her grandson a real favor, tell her to buy a measles shot here at the office. Shoes are okay. They suggest to the neighbors that you are a thoughtful mother, but they really won't do anything for his feet. He'll look dressed up for his first birthday party."

"What about his arches? His feet are just round blobs of fat with no arches that I can see."

"Arches will develop if they are going to. If his parents have flat feet, he will grow up to have flat feet. You may even make the tendency worse if you put him in shoes that are not pliable. Moccasins would be best if you feel you must have him shod."

"Why do all children wear shoes?"

"Tradition, habit, cement, and sharp objects. Protection is about the only reason for shoes."

"Well, she's probably going to get some, so what do I tell her?"

"Very soft ones, with the toe end roomy so he can wiggle and exercise his toes. High-laced shoes do not support the ankles particularly, but they are harder to pull off than low shoes."

"Tennis shoes okay?"

"Sure. Just make sure there is wiggle room. Remember, when he is two years old he will look knock-kneed and flat-footed. All babies do. Eventually the foot ligaments and the long tendons from the calf strengthen and the arch becomes an arch if he is going to have an arch—no matter what shoes you put on him."

"I'll try to tell her."

"You may get *her* to believe this, but shoe salesmen believe that they need stiff, high-laced shoes."

New Wives' Tale: If the floor is fairly clean, your toddler does not need to wear shoes.

"If the baby missed one DPT shot, start all over."

"The baby is eighteen months old. I'm all mixed up on his shots. He had one DPT and triple polio drops at six weeks, then we moved. He had another along with the drops at five months. Then he had a cold or diarrhea and they wouldn't give him the next shot and drops. We started again at nine months and he had his second in that series at ten months. Now the clinic says we must start again. He gets a fever and a sore arm each time. Do we have to do it all again?"

"Wow! Four times! He has more protection than most babies. From what I can gather from the research, he is safe from diphtheria, polio, whooping cough, and tetanus for about five to twenty years or more."

"Why do they start over?"

"I don't know. Maybe they don't keep up with the research. Special blood tests indicate that about 85 percent of babies are protected with just one shot plus polio drops. The second round increases that to 90 to 95 percent completely protected. The timing of a month or so between shots is just a convenience for memory's sake. One set a year would be okay, but we want to protect babies from whooping cough in the first few months; it's a big killer then."

"He's still alive."

"You were lucky. We still see these diseases, but almost exclusively in the unimmunized. The fever you mentioned is usually due to the dead whooping cough germs in the shot. Let me give him a booster in a smaller dose now and then again when he is five years old. We'll give him the measles shot, too."

New Wives' Tale: Give the baby three DPT shots as early in life as possible.

3

"You Never Outgrow Your Need for . . ."

The tired mother calls: "I am nursing my baby. He is full of gas and cramps and almost strangles on the phlegm in his throat."

The medical oracle announces: "He is getting too much milk or not enough and swallowing air. In either case you are transferring your nervousness to him; maybe you could get a calm friend to hold him up against you. Better yet, you'd better switch to the bottle and let your husband or a baby sitter feed him. Just take it easy, little mother; everything will be okay."

The scientist has spoken; there are no other options open. Thus abandoned by her medical adviser, the mother can get help only from friends, relatives, or the La Leche League. The latter may encourage her to continue nursing, but the baby's gas keeps rolling on. Just as an experiment, she tries a bottle of cow's milk, and the baby is much worse.

This suggests to her (if she has time to analyze it) that the baby is allergic to milk—or more specifically to the cow's milk *she* is drinking. She, on her own, tries a diet of no milk, ice cream, or cottage cheese for a few days and to her delight discovers her baby is a peaceful, happy, non-gas-former. (She also realizes her own gas problem has been reduced and she is not constipated any more.)

Her next problem is, of course, to figure out how to tell her doctor what she had done without upsetting him. It might be easier to switch doctors quietly. She is a little worried about the low-calcium diet, but her friendly druggist fixes her up with some nonprescription calcium pills.

What else could the doctor have said? All he was taught about milk in medical school was, "If it's there, it's good." A better truism would have been: "Cow's milk is for calves; human milk is for babies. If the breast-fed baby is full of gas, someone has adulterated the supply." Cows have to be careful about what they eat; so must humans. Garlic, onions, beans, and cabbage are just a few of the offenders that get from the mother's intestine into her milk and produce so much gas in the baby it tends to go sideways. It requires about 24 hours for food to go from mouth to anus, so a tuna fish sandwich a day might keep the baby floating off the mattress constantly. Cow's milk is just one offender of many.

Office visit: "My son is two years old. He had five ear infections in his first year, so his adenoids were removed. He was well for two months, then got a bad cold and started all over again. This time he had asthmatic bronchitis with it. He has been coughing and snorting since. We have to give him an antibiotic every four weeks. We give him vitamin C in big doses, but he is sickly. Have his adenoids grown back?"

Doctor: "Maybe the ear, nose, and throat doctor didn't get all the adenoid tissue out. Maybe he's anemic;

we'll check his blood. Maybe he's allergic; does he sleep with a feather pillow, wool blanket, or a dog or cat? Are you giving him vitamins?"

The doctor is stalling, because he really doesn't know why this otherwise healthy, well-fed child is sludged up with infection. His tonsils are somewhat enlarged, he looks pale, he has circles under his eyes, his eardrums look thickened, pink, and dull, and he keeps clearing his throat. His blood test shows a borderline anemia, so he is put on some iron tonic. An antibiotic is prescribed.

The child improves because of the antibiotic. The iron increases his appetite for meat, fruit, and vegetables. At about the same time, his milk intake decreases. (The appetite loss of the two-year-old is traditional; he may have developed an aversion to milk.) His health is credited to the antibiotic by the mother and to the correction of the anemia by the doctor. One week of increased intake of milk and ice cream while he was staying with grandmother is followed by a "cold," 102° fever, and pus draining from his ears. He is well now if he uses milk only on his cereal and drinks orange juice and water. His ear infections follow birthday parties where chocolate milk and ice cream are served.

Old Wives' Tale: "You'll die if you don't drink your milk."

"You told me if I stopped serving milk, ice cream, and cottage cheese to my son, his sniffing, snorting, throat clearing, coughing, and choking would clear up."

"I said it might be better."

"Well, he's been off the cow for ten days. The phlegm is almost gone. He's made a noise with every breath since birth, so we always knew he was okay. Now how do we tell? Last night his breathing was so quiet we had to hold a mirror up to his nose to see if he was still alive."

"It does take some getting used to. Is his color better? He was so pale the other day. He had circles under his eyes and he had stomach aches and headaches."

"Oh, yes. His cheeks are pink and he has no complaints. He seems to have more energy, too. He sleeps more restfully."

"I'm glad to hear it's working out so well and so easily. You might use a little milk on his cereal or give some ice cream occasionally; maybe he can tolerate some."

"But I'm so worried, doctor. Is he going to die?"

"What?"

"Won't he die if he doesn't drink milk?"

"Did your mother tell you that?"

"Yes. I hate milk. My mother used to stand over us at mealtime, point at us, and shout, 'You'll die if you don't drink milk!' "

New Wives' Tale: Mothers don't know everything.

"If you can't eat your dinner, at least drink your milk" is the cheer echoed in homes throughout our country, Canada, and Europe—wherever there is a cow nearby. We were all taught this in hygiene and nutrition classes at elementary, high, and college level, and even in medical school. "A quart of milk a day is ideal," they told us, "but it might be safe to let this dip to a pint a day for the two- to four-year-old whose appetite is off." But rapid growth of teeth and bones makes a large intake of calcium a necessity; and where does the child get calcium if he is not drinking his milk? Milk has protein (for muscles) and carbohydrates and fat (for energy); what could be more ideal? Look how big the calf gets!

In our nutrition classes in medical school we took notes, copied the chart (four basic foods: meat, grains, fruit and vegetables, and dairy products—courtesy of the American Dairy Council)—and passed the exams. Armed with these facts, we new doctors went into practice to straighten out the world. It soon became painfully obvious that what we had learned as basic universal food facts did not fit every situation.

Phone call: "I'm desperate. My sweet daughter is two years old and I would like to toilet train her. Her stools are big and hard. They cause cracking and bleeding. This hurts her so she refused to use the toilet; now the stools come out in small hard pieces in her sleep or at odd times in the day in her underwear."

The doctor immediately forms a mental picture of a rigid, demanding home trying to coerce a normal, somewhat defiant two-year-old, who responds with passive-aggressive withholding. He tries to get the mother to back off.

"Laxatives?"

"Yes, they soften them but I don't want to rely on them."

"Extra water?"

"Yes, she loves to drink milk, water, and juice, but she just urinates more and the stools remain firm."

"Could she stay with a relative for a while? Maybe you two need a rest from each other," says the doctor, trying not to put too much obvious blame on the mother. The child goes to Aunt Mary's for two weeks and has no trouble except that she almost falls in the toilet bowl once, as the seat size is unfamiliar. Her stools soften up, she goes fearlessly into the bathroom and seems to be more active and cheerful. I'm sure you have already guessed that Aunt Mary is on a diet of meat and fruit and eats nothing white—the traditional high-carbohydrate, high-calorie foods.

We were told in medical school that harsh laxatives were dangerous and the patient might develop a dependency. Roughage foods and bulk laxatives were the answer, but the professors were loath to discourage milk ingestion because *they* had been taught that we all need the calcium and protein that milk provides. When milk hits the stomach, it is curdled by the acid. This chunk moves through the intestines and becomes drier and harder as the moisture is absorbed from it. By the time it reaches the rectum it is a large, rubbery ball that may defy expulsion. Most of us do not enjoy digital digging into the rectum of a frightened three-year-old. Magnesia salts and enemas may provide temporary relief, but how much easier it is to avoid the whole problem by monitoring what food goes into the upper end! All white foods (with the exception of cauliflower) are considered constipating; in addition, white foods are virtually devoid of iron. The two- to four-year-old child is a special problem because (1) he may be cutting teeth and hates to chew, (2) his parents are trying to toilet train him, and his attention is drawn to his elimination, (3) his appetite is at a low ebb, and (4) he whines a great deal, which might make his throat dry. The milk feels so good going down. His parents encourage milk ingestion because they have heard that it is "good" for him and "at least he is eating something." He has one large, hard, dry stool which cracks the anal lining, so he decides he will never have another movement. The longer he holds it, the harder it gets. His bloat discourages his appetite. Yet he is still able to swallow some milk and ice cream. Then the harassed pediatrician has to straighten him out and/or dig him out.

"My four-year-old is fine except that she goes grunt-grunt only two times a week. Is this bad? Grandmother says it's bad because it hurts the brain and she will have convulsions or go crazy. I know that's not true; or is it?"

"I haven't heard that old wives' tale for two months. She's probably been watching those laxative ads on TV. 'Irregularity' is supposed to make grandparents snarly just when the grandchildren are coming for a pleasant weekend visit. Consistency, not frequency, seems to be the important criterion for normalcy. If it is comfortably expellable, it is okay. If it is a big rock and you need a stick to break it up to flush it, better cut out the white foods, especially dairy products."

We had a professor in medical school who told it like it was: "The only contraindication to the use of mineral oil seems to be a slippery pavement." Most constipated people know about roughage foods, but forget to cut down on white foods, milk, and cheese.

Phone call, 7:00 P.M.: "You have to do something. Our mealtimes are deteriorating into screaming, crying, food-throwing fights. I had always looked forward to the happy end of the day; the picture of the tired but happy family gathered at the festive board, sharing experiences, joined together by my tasty, nutritious food is an ideal I can't pull off. We are all so tense we can hardly eat; our stomachs are in knots. The kids pick at their food. My husband sees the fruit of his hard labor lying on the plates, so he force-feeds the children, saying something about 'growing up to be big and strong.'

Of course they throw it all up, and then even the dog won't touch it. Please help!"

A doctor who has the identical problem at *his* house may respond with some anger-provoking putdown like, "Don't serve brussels sprouts and cauliflower until they are older," or "Feed them before the old man gets home," or "Don't let them nibble at 5:00 P.M. if dinner is at 6:00."

The doctor's training allows him only one generalization: "nutritious food served in pleasant surroundings." No one ever told him how *much* food, probably because no one *knows* how much to serve. Parents become used to the baby's huge appetite in his first year and are unprepared for the drop off after age one-and-a-half to three years when the child grows only three inches in a year (ten inches in the first year) and gains only three to four pounds in a year (fifteen pounds gained in the first year).

Depressed, the mother broils a hamburger patty apiece and commands, "Don't eat it." They do. She has stumbled on a food truism not usually taught in nutrition class: serve small amounts that will be consumed and let the child ask the cook for more. (The child is put in the position of asking the mother for seconds; the parent is again put in the role of being needed. She also discovers that if less milk is served, the children eat more of the food on their plates.)

Office visit: "John is seven years old now and it's time he stopped wetting the bed. He has good daytime control, but he soaks the bed almost every night. He was dry most of the summer but started to wet again when school started. Is this related to some psychological pressure at school? We try not to scold him, but he seems so hurt when he cannot control it. He doesn't dare stay overnight with friends."

Doctor (after urinalysis and X-ray studies): "Everything is structurally all right. Is it a family trait?"

Mother: "Under pressure his father admitted he wet the bed a few times." (The paternal grandmother remembers it as more like a few times a night until age thirteen.)

Doctor: "Sounds like school is too much for him."

Mother (later): "He hasn't wet since we moved and he comes home to eat his lunch. Maybe it's the milk he drinks with the school lunch. He ate some watermelon the other night and he was dry, but after some sherbet last night he flooded the bed."

I know a boy who drank no milk because he wet the bed whenever he did. He continued this from age five until adolescence, when he seemed to outgrow it. When he was twelve years old he broke his leg while skiing. As his doctor, I was apprehensive, as I thought the X ray he needed would reveal the folly of this low-calcium diet. The orthopedic surgeon I called in to treat him not only found the fracture but commented on the appearance of the bone. "Shows he's drinking his milk," he said. *Then* I told him about the milk-poor diet. He was astounded; he, as I, had memorized the Dairy Council's chart of the basic foods. (Even excessive genital interest could be diminished by withdrawing milk from the diet if milk had been causing the child's bottom to itch.)

Office visit: "Check his blood. He looks terrible: circles under his eyes, pale, tired, stomach aches and headaches and irritable. He snorts every six seconds; I timed it. My mother-in-law *knows* I'm doing something wrong. Does he need vitamins or iron, or both? Maybe it's worms."

Doctor (a little miffed because *he* wanted to suggest the blood count): "Okay, okay, we'll check it." Hemoglobin test is 12 grams. "A little low but not bad. Why not try some iron anyway?"

A month later the blood test is 13.5 grams, normal, but the pallor and pains and tiredness are still present.

Doctor (through clenched teeth): "Hold it. I was looking through his chart and now recall that he was fussy and colicky as a baby when he was on milk alone. Why don't you stop dairy products for a while?"

Mother: "But won't he waste away if he doesn't have milk? What about teeth and bones?"

Phone call (three weeks later): "He looks and acts great. Stays up late. Gets up early. A regular pest, but at least he's cheerful."

This condition, called *tension-fatigue syndrome,* has now joined the ranks of accredited diseases with reproducible symptoms directly related to ingestion of certain foods, usually milk. (Chocolate, eggs, wheat, or pork may also be responsible.) Dark half-circles of the lower eyelids, pallor (with or without accompanying anemia), headaches, stomach aches, fatigue, irritability, muscle cramps, and a characteristic "zonking" noise give away the condition. This sound is produced by the victim as he attempts to clear the excess mucus clinging to the back of his nasal passages and palate; he feels as if a bunch of rubber bands are stuck back there and he cannot release them. He may not sneeze or rub his nose, the hallmark of an inhalation allergy. He may have frequent bacterial (mucus is green or yellow) upper respiratory or sinus or ear infections aggravated by colds. After three weeks of no milk, ice cream, or cottage cheese, the symptoms all clear up and he can smell things for the first time in his life.

"My child gets anemic all the time. His blood and bone marrow have been tested, the doctors have ruled out TB, rheumatic fever, nephritis, and bleeding ulcers and polyps in his intestines. He gets dewormed every six months but we can't get his hemoglobin to stay above 11.5 grams (12.5 to 14 is normal). Iron medicine helps but then the blood count slips back again."

The doctor scans his brain for some answer no one has thought of. "Does he take a lot of aspirin because of headaches?" Maybe this mother hovers over the child and he gets headaches, just like the doctor is getting now because he can't think of the answer. "Aspirin can burn holes in the stomach lining, regardless of what the Bufferin people say."

"No."

"I've got it! Bloody noses?"

"No."

"How about an allergy to some food?" Allergy is always a safe bet; it's vague, sneaky, and can affect any organ of the body.

"I won't buy it. No sneezing or wheezing."

Then the doctor recalls a journal article about microscopic bleeding from the intestinal lining following ingestion of common allergenic foods, notably milk, eggs, pork, and nuts. "You've tried everything else."

The patient is placed on iron, and dairy products are proscribed. In a month the hemoglobin value is up a whole gram for the first time in years.

The common milk anemia is due to the excessive ingestion of milk plus an accompanying inadequate intake of meat, vegetables, and fruit. Occasionally a diet adequate in iron-bearing foods is not enough to compensate for the loss of blood from thousands of microscopic leaks from intestinal capillaries. It is hard to believe that nice, clean milk could be a nutritional enemy.

So the child is better but the mother comes back with a zinger. "Okay, so milk is the culprit. Won't his bones and teeth turn to gelatin because of the low calcium in his diet?"

An old doctor might be able to remember rickets from the old days. "Soft bones are due to lack of vitamin D, not calcium. Years ago when babies developed rickets, they were drinking plenty of milk, so calcium ingestion was not the answer. Vitamin D acts as an enzyme to pick up what calcium is available in the intestines and get it to the bones and teeth. Most milk has D in it now so maybe a vitamin D supplement would be worthwhile now that he is off milk."

A young doctor might not have such a smart answer but at least would know where to look it up.

This brings up an interesting point. What happens to growing children in countries with no cows or goats? One must assume they have a low-calcium diet, but apparently running about naked in the sun gives them enough vitamin D to permit maximum utilization of the small amounts of calcium in their diets. The Eskimos get vitamin D from the fish they eat.

In the last ten years nutrition research has discovered that about 75 to 90 percent of blacks, Orientals, and Indians (East and West) are unable to break down lactose, the milk sugar, because of the absence of the intestinal enzyme lactase. This double sugar (a disaccharide) is unabsorbable, so it remains in the intestinal tract; there, bacteria ferment it, producing gas, cramps, and usually diarrhea in its victims, who think they might have the flu or dysentery. Imagine the reluctance of these peoples to trust Americans or believe in our foreign policy when the skim milk powder we send them tears out their insides. The package reads, "From your friends in the United States." It is reported that the recipients use the powder as whitewash for their huts and fences. These people who are lactase-deficient constitute most of the population of Asia, Africa, South America, and Mexico. Many of those living on the Mediterranean shores are lacking this enzyme, a fact which must also account for their use of cheese, yogurt, and buttermilk (rather than whole milk), as these are devoid of lactose. But people on a dairy-free diet have no reported deficiencies in tooth or bone structure, so their calcium is obviously derived from other sources.

Phone call: "Do you treat acne? My adolescent is a pimply mess. He washes with soap and a washcloth, uses a sunlamp, uses tetracycline which helps some, and pats on a variety of lotions from the druggist and the dermatologist. What now? Is it bad thoughts and self-abuse?"

Doctor: "Wow, you've tried it all. What does the dermatologist suggest next?"

Parent: "Needling the big ones and injecting cortisone. Can an allergy do this?"

Doctor: "We are not supposed to believe it is related, but why don't you try cutting out milk and chocolate?"

Parent (a month later): "His face is much better but not cured."

(Rule: If something goes wrong with the body, and it is not infection, trauma, worms, or sleeping with the dog, try cutting out milk.)

Milk is a good food but not a perfect food. At least 15 to 20 percent of the population should not touch it, or should curtail its intake. Dairy-consuming countries have a higher than average incidence of vascular problems (strokes and heart attacks).

I realize I should spend more time and energy in attacking the evils of soft drinks, junk food, candy, and rich desserts, but the dairy advertisements suggest that survival is dependent on milk consumption, a patent lie. The public is made to feel guilty if large volumes of milk are not ingested daily. Some people feel it is immoral to steal milk from the cow.

New Wives' Tale: Caution: Milk may be a hazard to your health.

4

"Nothing Goes in the Mouth but Food and Drink"

Old Wives' Tale: "If you have breasts, you should nurse your baby."

"*Should* I nurse my baby?"

If a mother asks this question, it usually means she has negative feelings about nursing, and pushing her into it may not be the best for all concerned.

"What do you want to do?" I say evasively.

"I don't know. You're the expert. You tell me."

"You put me in a difficult position. If I say you *have* to and it is unsuccessful, you will feel guilty. My real job is to give you the options, let you decide, but then encourage and support your choice. You're a woman and a mother, but because you express some doubts, it may not work. But now that I've said that, now you will assume I have some doubts about your ability, and that will make your doubts worse. Stop! Look, I'll encourage you like I'm supposed to. You can do it and I'll help. Nurse him as frequently as possible, but for only a few minutes at a time. Maybe I can get the nurses to bring him out when he's hungry and not when they want to bring him, like every four hours."

"Passing the buck. You guys are sure wishy-washy."

"A better phrase might be permissive within limits. There are many right ways to do things. Breastfeeding is one. Your baby is two days old, this hospital allows a modified rooming-in, feeding-on-demand schedule, and the nurses are sympathetic to breastfeeding. Why don't you try?"

In the hospital, the first attempt at nursing often goes like this:

(Here he comes for the 10:00 P.M. feeding. I can hear him screaming down the hall. Maybe if his mouth is open big enough he will glom onto my breast and get the milk started; I can feel a tingling there now. Come on, milk! Come on, Mark!)

"Yes, I'm Mrs. Starheim. Yes, that's Mark." *(Quick—get him over here. Aim him. He missed! I smashed into his cheek, but he's turning his head.)*

A protective reflex allows a normal baby to direct his mouth to any object touching his cheek. The harder one tries to push his face onto the breast, the more he turns away. Ever so gently let the nipple brush by his lips, chin, or cheek and he will turn and lock on.

(Oh, boy! He got it. Ouch! Not so hard. How sweet he is. Now I'm getting a menstrual cramp.)

Most women notice uterine cramps if a baby is nursing well. This is one of the benefits of nursing: the uterus reverts to normal size more quickly in nursing mothers. Apparently there is some hormone release that stimulates the uterine muscles to contract.

(Here comes the nurse again.) "Time's up. Not too long at first or your nipples will get sore and cracked."

(That's great. We'll make a fine team. And for a while there I didn't think of a single other problem and I

forgot to be depressed. Having a baby is good therapy for having a baby.)

The depression that most women suffer two to five days after delivery is a mixture of hormone withdrawal, end of the intrauterine job and its psychological support, plus sudden realization of a new untested role, motherhood, and fifteen years of the PTA. Society has evolved the gift-giving, the homage-paying, and the various supports offered to the new mother because they are stylized sanity savers.

Research indicates that the breasts will do what they are going to do, nurse or not. It appears to be genetically arranged. The fat content and the amount of elastic tissue will determine the outcome.

(Here he comes again, screaming. How can he get anything from me if I haven't eaten anything for twelve hours?)

They do. Mothers on a starvation diet can still manufacture milk. The sugar, calcium, and protein stored through the body will be mobilized to fill the need. Fluid lack would be the chief immediate concern. If a woman is not used to drinking extra fluid she will find it difficult to produce milk. A good rule: if fairly dilute urine is being excreted by the nursing mother three or four times a day, she is probably drinking enough; the same rule would apply to the baby. Some women can drink a large glass of water at nursing time and feel the milk fill their breasts.

(Now he's quiet, busily sucking. I think he swallowed something. I'll just nuzzle his head. How soft he is. He smells good.)

"How about when I get home?"

"Is your husband helpful and sympathetic?"

"He's pretty good, but I do have to spell things out

for him. He's not too intuitive. How can he help? He's built differently than I."

"He's supposed to help with meals and housework unless he's a complete chauvinist. You can get involved with the La Leche League and both of you should be members of the Association for Childbirth Education; I'm surprised you don't already belong. They are very supportive."

"What about my diet later? How much milk should I drink?"

"Probably, if you eat some meat, fruit, vegetable, and cereal or bread, you'll get enough of everything so you won't need vitamins. Your obstetrician will feel safer if you continue on the vitamins and iron you took during your pregnancy. Don't eat chocolate, fish, beans, cabbage, garlic, onions, or the gas-forming foods; they will get in your milk and give Mark gas cramps."

"I hate cow's milk. How much do I *have* to drink?"

"None. Even if you don't drink a quart of milk a day, your body will be able to manufacture breast milk in abundance. If you have a balanced diet, you will get all you need without it. Do you like beer? Sometimes a quart of beer a day gives you fluids and provides some tranquility; if you are stoned, however, you may not be able to find the baby at feeding time. Give it a try; I'll be your rooting section."

"Okay. Sounds like a lot of work."

"Now that's the point. If you are depressed and discouraged, it won't be fun. If you don't think it's fun, it won't work. Motivation is essential. I've had some patients who adopted newborns and were able to nurse. It took a week or so to really get the milk up to a satisfactory amount, but they did it. Apparently the sucking stimulated the hypothalamus in the brain to get the lactogenic hormone to flow. This hormone makes the milk glands function. Try it; you'll like it."

"Okay. If you don't mind a worried mother calling a lot."

New Wives' Tale: Nursing depends on what's in your head, not on your chest.

"Boil water, milk, bottles, and nipples before the baby uses them."

"By the way, when can I stop boiling the nipples and bottles for the baby? He's six months old now and puts everything in his mouth, even his toes, and I can't boil those."

"Oops, I'm sorry. I thought everyone knew that boiling bottles and formula was no longer necessary."

"Won't he get germs or diarrhea or something?"

"Sure they get germs, but if you're not a typhoid carrier, what he gets are nice germs. Someone did some testing and discovered that within a few hours of birth a baby has been 'colonized' all through his intestinal tract with all the usual bacteria that we adults have."

"Ugh! Why am I doing all this extra work?"

"Years ago when sanitation was at a minimum, many people carried about many of those dysentery bacteria and boiling was lifesaving. Sometimes the outdoor privy was close to and draining into the well. Some well water has nitrates which will oxidize the baby's hemoglobin and make him turn a muddy, blue color."

"Tap water is okay?"

"If you can drink it, so can your baby. I don't mean you should be slovenly. Get all the milk curds out with a bottle brush, then use hot water and soap. The water in the automatic dishwasher is plenty hot enough. I read of a study done on the bacteria population of infant formulas. A mother was using powdered Similac and boiled water, a combination that should have been virtually bacteria-free. They discovered massive bacterial pollution. When the researchers reviewed her mixing technique, they found she was leveling the milk powder in the measuring cup with her finger instead of a sterilized knife. The baby did not suffer any upset because he was getting friendly finger germs. But too many nice germs can be upsetting, so some cleanliness is advisable. Babies need to be exposed to a few environmental hazards. I'm impressed with the survival rate of the many babies bathed in the Ganges River."

"Ugh, again. Just dump it in the bottle and then into him?"

"Right. The fastest way is to pour the concentrated milk into the bottle, then run the same amount of hot water from the tap, screw on the nipple, and stick it into his mouth. It takes about 25 seconds from hunger cry to first swallow."

New Wives' Tale: The baby needs to get familiar with the family bacteria.

"Heat the baby's milk to 90° or so before feeding."

"I'm sorry to call you like it's an emergency, but I'm so worried. My husband just fed our four-day-old baby a bottle of cold milk!"

"Steady now. Did the baby drink it?"

"Sure; he was so hungry he slugged it down. Will he vomit or get colic?"

"What's he doing right now?"

"Sleeping like a baby."

"Then I would assume there is no problem."

"Won't he get bad cramps?"

"No. Somebody did a study of newborn bottle-fed babies and discovered that about half would accept cold milk and suffer no ill effects. The other half of the group wouldn't even drink it. They were either not hungry enough or wanted warmed milk."

"You mean I don't need to warm up his milk?"

"Maybe he's an easy-going baby and doesn't care. Maybe he trusts you so much that he thinks whatever you do is okay. Maybe he thinks all babies get cold milk."

"Little does he know what a tough father he's got."

"I suppose because breast milk is served at body temperature, we have all assumed bottle milk must be at the same temperature. But a baby's body warms it up as soon as he takes it. If you happen to have warm milk around, it makes a good culture medium for bacteria. I did a little experiment on our children because they always wanted a 2:00 A.M. feeding and I was in charge of the 11:00 P.M. to 6:00 A.M. problems. I put a bottle of cold milk at the bedside when I went to bed so by the time the baby announced his hunger pain, the chill would be off. So you might try a compromise."

"It sounds a little mean."

New Wives' Tale: If a baby drinks the milk, its temperature is probably okay.

"Put the baby on a schedule or he will soon rule the house."

"I'm trying to work out a four-hour feeding schedule, but the baby won't cooperate very well. Sometimes he sleeps for six hours, and I hate to wake him up. Then in late afternoon and early evening he seems to want to nibble every two hours and I go nuts listening to him cry for the two more hours before the next scheduled feeding. Will I spoil him if I feed him sooner than every four hours?"

"I think he's trying to tell you something. Few babies are cooperative about being hungry at four-hour intervals. The liquid milk is moved out of the stomach in one and a half to two hours, so he might need to be fed every two hours. Hopefully he will nurse every two hours in the daytime and sleep all night. Most babies cry when they are hungry, and they have no respect for the wishes of the household. He's hungry because he's growing fast. If he continued at this rate, by the time he was ten years old he would be twenty feet tall. Obviously he'll slow down, but not for a while yet."

"You mean he can be hungry in an hour or two?"

"Sure. It's just liquid. I would suggest you feed him every two hours."

"I'll be feeding him all day."

"Yes, but if you get his quota for the twenty-four hours in him in the twelve daylight hours, he—and you—can sleep all night. That seems to be the best schedule. By the way, you don't set your alarm for 2:00 A.M., wake him up, and feed him, do you?"

"Well . . . I . . . uh. . . ."

"Come on. A mother is supposed to be self-sacrificing, but you're making this baby into a hair shirt. I'm told that Dutch babies never cry at night—or at least are not fed at night—and thus have learned that crying for food at that time is futile. Some argue that there is a genetic memory for sleeping through the night, but it may also mean that the baby is put upstairs and the parents sleep downstairs out of earshot. The baby may thus consume huge amounts the next day to get ready for the next long night. If you feed yours consistently at night he will learn that he is supposed to eat in the middle of the night. You reward him for awakening at 2:00 A.M."

"But he's so hungry then."

"Try to cheat him a little bit. Every few nights give him a little less milk at that feeding. He might learn to eat more during the day."

"Yeah. Sure."

"He's a guest in your house. Get him used to the activity-inactivity fluctuations of *your* household."

As the weeks go by, however, no matter what method is used, the baby on a demand or rigid schedule will gradually adjust to the rhythm of the household and sleep when his parents do. Forceful readjustment of the baby's feeding pattern usually leads to frustration. If a mother tries to arouse a new baby for a feeding in two hours when his locked-in pattern demands a four-hour deep sleep, she will be faced with stubborn, unassailable negativism. She might get some cooperation at three hours and forty-five minutes, however.

New Wives' Tale: Feed a baby when he is hungry, but try to teach him to be hungry during the day.

"Babies need extra water."

"Between feedings I try to give the baby a drink of water but he just chokes and spits it out. Occasionally he loses the previous meal. Don't tell me I have to give it rectally."

"It is true that up to six months of age the infant's kidneys do not concentrate urine well and hence do not tolerate dehydration well."

"But how do I get down the fluid that he needs if he won't take it? How about apple juice?"

"Maybe he doesn't need extra fluid. The formula you

use is almost 90 percent water. A rule we use goes something like this: If a baby gets about two ounces of fluid for each pound of weight in the twenty-four hour period, he gets enough fluid. If the air temperature gets above 90° to 100° he probably needs about 10 percent more fluid. At his present ten pounds he should get at least twenty ounces of fluid a day. Are you getting that in?"

"Oh, yes. He gets almost a quart a day."

"How about his urine? Three or four times a day?"

"Are you kidding? He swims six times a day."

"No problem. If it gets hot, or he vomits, or he has diarrhea, just add a little water to the formula."

New Wives' Tale: If a baby is urinating three or four times a day, he is probably getting enough fluid.

"Give the baby extra water if he has a diaper rash."

"My baby has a terrible rash in the diaper area. We are giving extra water, but he just wets more."

"Why are you doing that?"

"Aren't you supposed to?"

"Water is useful for thirst. Actually some diaper rashes are made worse with fluid. Does he smell of ammonia in the morning?"

"Wow! It drives me out of the room. I was thinking of using the diapers to cut the dirt and grease on the windows. Doesn't water dilute the ammonia?"

"Somewhat. Actually more fluid just makes more urine available to manufacture the ammonia. Concentrated urine is not the cause. The cause is a bacteria in the diaper that changes urine into ammonia."

"I wash the diapers. Should I change soap?"

"It's a tough germ. Boiling and bleaching won't help. Put the diapers out in the sunshine."

"This is Oregon, remember?"

"Okay, use disposable diapers or put one ounce of vinegar in the second of four diapers when you put him to bed at night."

"Vinegar?"

"Yes. It's cheap and acidic; this counteracts the alkalinity of the ammonia. But cut down on the fluid. If he urinates three or four times a day, he's getting enough fluid."

"He is swimming eight times a day."

"One mother told me she cut a hole in the mattress, lined it with plastic, and put a bucket underneath. The rash disappeared, but one night the baby almost did, too. Another mother coated her baby's bottom with a heavy ointment and plastered strips of Saran Wrap on top of this. The urine no longer hit the skin and the rash cleared."

New Wives' Tale: If a diaper rash is due to irritating urine, remove the irritant.

"Colic is caused by a nervous mother."

"Please help me. This two-week-old baby is driving me wild. How can something this small turn our house completely upside down? I feed him and he screams; I don't feed him and he screams. Is this colic?"

"Any screaming that is not caused by hunger is colic. Maybe that's a scare word to you. Some call it 'wind,' which doesn't have such a frightening connotation."

"Okay, it's wind. What do I do about it? I'm a wreck. I read your book and have made the nipple holes so big he almost drowns. I've put him on his right side. I burp him after every ounce. I feed him every hour and a half. I've used a glycerine suppository to help him pass his wind, but he just goes on bellowing. I can almost sympathize with those people who batter their children. My mother-in-law says I'm nervous. Who wouldn't be?"

"You're way ahead of me. You've tried all my suggestions. One doctor said it was an 'immature intestinal tract' and the baby is crampy because he has to eat so much to prevent hunger pains that he gets bloated. It would be the same distress that you and I would feel if we ate six spaghetti dinners in twelve hours."

"I have to feed him, don't I?"

"Yes. Anyone gets tense, anxious, and frustrated if he tries to do something for someone but only seems to make the situation worse. One of our children was an overreactor. I can remember him screaming after eating at 2:00 A.M. I found that if I put one little finger in his mouth and the other little finger in his rectum, he was content to suck and pass wind as long as I would stand there. I would sneak back into bed and just get to sleep when he would begin again. I'd rush back to him and try to remember which finger went to which end. I finally opted for a sedative."

"I'll take the sedative, thank you."

"I'll call your drugstore. It's quite a safe barbiturate. Maybe you could give it with the feeding just prior to the bad time. If it makes him worse, that's supposed to mean he's hyperactive."

"It's bad all the time."

"Give a little with each feeding. Just enough to quiet the cramps without knocking him out completely."

"Maybe *I* should take some."

"You're okay. Your response is a normal reaction to his overawareness of his digestion. If you don't feel comfortable when he settles down, let me examine him and talk to you. If he still doesn't settle down, we'll try some soybean milk."

New Wives' Tale: A colicky baby makes a parent tense, which upsets the baby, which upsets the parents which . . . etc.

"If a baby has diarrhea, give him boiled skimmed milk."

"My baby vomited three days ago and has had five watery green stools a day ever since. He is fussy, crampy, his eyes are sunken, and he seems so listless. I'm giving him boiled skimmed milk and Kaopectate, but it goes right through him. How do I constipate him?"

"You're doing the right things, except I thought everyone knew now that feeding boiled milk was dangerous."

"I thought that made it more digestible and constipating."

"Up to a point. The boiling concentrates the milk and this sodium-rich fluid is absorbed and only makes the dehydration worse. We occasionally see convulsions in babies when the sodium gets too high. Don't boil it. Skimmed milk is okay, but add a little water to each bottle, maybe two ounces of water to each four ounces of milk. Babies lose more water than salt."

"I guess I'm a failure. I've always heard that boiled skimmed milk was the best."

"It's too strong unless diluted, and plain water doesn't have any minerals. Somewhere in between is best."

New Wives' Tale: If a baby has diarrhea, call the doctor; he may know something you don't.

"If a child won't eat, you must force-feed him."

"My girl is ten months old and she refuses to eat. Is she teething? Maybe she has a sore throat, but she has no fever. What should I do?"

"I'll look at her throat, but sore throats at her age are usually accompanied by fever. Tell me how you feed her."

"The usual way. She sits at the table and I spoon-feed her—or try to. She just clamps her jaws tight and shakes her head. I pry her mouth open and poke the spoon in, but I usually get it right back again. She screams and I get mad. She'll get anemic, won't she, if she doesn't get any solids?"

"That's true, but it takes a while. You say you have her sit at your table while you eat?"

"Yes."

"Does she pick up food with her fingers and put the bits into her mouth?"

"Well, she tries. But it's so messy. I slap her hands and give her a spoon. She throws that on the floor and the fight begins."

"I think she's trying to tell you something. She sees you feed yourself and she wants to imitate."

"Why doesn't she use the spoon? I do."

"She's not ready for that. Fingers were made before forks, they say."

"Not hers. Why are children so messy? If it isn't at one end, it's the other."

"Come on; make it fun. Give her a boiled carrot or some soft cooked hamburger or ground-up luncheon meat. We used to mix cooked oatmeal and applesauce together for our kids' breakfast. They would scoop this up with their fingers and get it all in their mouths with almost no spill. Scrambled egg can be neat. Lunch might be a peanut butter and jam sandwich. This age often feels they have to kill the food by squeezing before they eat it; then they smash it on the table. If it's not moving, then they'll eat it."

"Ugh!"

"Really. They have to go through this. Don't fight her, join her. Dump some soft-cooked chunks of food in front of her and turn your back. Having a dog around to eat up the leftovers may help. Don't watch her if it bothers you. And be sure to cut down on the milk so she will be hungry enough to gobble up the solids. No peanuts or raw diced carrots."

"When will she use the spoon?"

"When her nervous system tells her she is ready. If you force it on her, it'll take her longer to use it. You have to make good adult table manners look like fun, then she'll eventually imitate you."

"I'll never get her married off."

New Wives' Tale: Learning waits on motivation which waits on maturation.

"If a child eats properly, he won't get sick."

"My children eat meat and fruit and even some vegetables, both cooked and raw, but they are constantly sick with colds and coughs. They get sunshine, vitamins, iron supplements, vitamin C up to 1,000 milligrams, plenty of sleep and exercise. What have I left out?"

"Love and prayer should complete the list. Someone did a study and found that anemic children had twice the average incidence of respiratory infections. We could check that out."

"Even if they're taking iron?"

"Some rapid growers get anemic because they cannot absorb enough iron to keep up with their needs, but that's unusual when extra iron is being taken."

"The in-laws see these snotty-nosed kids and think I'm a lousy mother."

"Two allergies come to mind which may explain the problem. Repeated respiratory infections almost surely mean allergy. Milk is a common food that may create a chronic phlegm condition, which makes people more susceptible to colds and sinusitis. Do they zonk?"

"You mean that horrible sniffling, snorting sound?"

"Yes. You might stop dairy products for a while."

"I'm way ahead of you. I've heard you lecture on the evils of milk and have already tried eliminating it. That helped but they still sound clogged up."

"House dust, mold, and animal allergies might be responsible. I'll give you an allergy check list and if that doesn't help, we'll have to do some skin testing."

New Wives' Tale: If one eats properly, he may still get sick for other reasons.

"A child should learn to eat what's on his plate."

"As you know, my son is hyperactive and a nibbler. He sneaks handfuls of sugar out of the sugar bowl, and a dozen cookies are gone in seventeen minutes. The dentist is screaming. The tougher I get, the more he does it. Today I found half a loaf of bread in his pillow-case. He's very thin, so I guess he needs it, but how do I get him to eat the right things? Should he have vitamins?"

"The brain has to have a constant supply of sugar in order to function. One authority found that the brain accounts for 25 percent of the body's metabolism. Since he has this sugar craving, the hyperactive child's brain must burn it up faster."

"I can't let him eat sugar all day."

"He can get energy from good, nutritious food. Some mothers compromise, so they don't have to fight. If a child is thirsty, you let him drink. If he is hungry, you let him eat."

"Sounds permissive."

"Yes, but permissive within limits. Make a rule about *what* he eats, but let him decide *when* he needs to eat. Have a bowl on the kitchen table with a sign, 'Charlie's Bowl.' The bowl is full of grapes, raisins, dried apricots, nuts, pepperoni, chipped beef, salami, and cheese. You might have a few crackers and an apple or orange in there, too. He's allowed to eat anything that's in the bowl at any time, and you keep it filled. He's happy because he maintains his blood sugar at acceptable levels, and you're supposed to be happy because he is eating good food—meat and fruit."

"It doesn't seem right, somehow."

New Wives' Tale: Don't make rules you can't enforce; don't enforce rules that make no sense.

"If parents eat the proper foods, so will the children."

"I'm a pretty good cook and serve balanced meals to the family. We have much variety, but each of the three children *and* my husband have some strange likes and dislikes. It doesn't make sense. Why should the ten-year-old refuse to eat carrots unless they're raw? I love carrots but she acts as if they are poisonous. She's not allergic because she ate them as a baby and they agreed with her."

"Some people don't like carrots."

"Another child hates gravy and drinks gallons of juice. The third one hates meat, and when he does eat some he has to shred it up into its individual fibrils. My husband loves to nibble: cookies, peanuts, potato chips, eclairs. He never gets fat. I love vinegar dressing, pickles, and sour food. What am I doing wrong?"

"Nothing, except expecting to change peoples' life styles. You can't bend your elbow backwards. We are just learning about enzymes and body chemistry because science is able to measure these things. We all have different ways of using and eliminating various chemicals; maybe you have odd kidneys that need to have more acidic chemicals to function properly. Hyperactive people need more sugar because the brain cannot metabolize fat as an energy source. Maybe the meat hater can tolerate only so much protein because too much overloads some enzyme system. Maybe some people need more vitamin C for health than what nutritionists are willing to admit."

"What do I do with *my* family?"

"Teach them to be courteous to one another and accept each other's idiosyncrasies as endearing traits; avoid the offending foods, but make sure they all get some meat, fruit or vegetable, and grain almost every day. Some dairy products are okay, but don't emphasize white foods. Especially discourage white flour, cakes, sugar on everything, salt on everything, and rich desserts."

New Wives' Tale: Eat some meat and fruit every day and you will be close to a reasonable diet.

"Children will eat if mealtime is calm and the food attractively served."

"I know you're just a pediatrician, but can you suggest something for me to try at meals to make it a happy time? I serve small portions and little or no milk as you suggest and that helps. Our problem is Kevin, who is a little hyperactive and tends to nibble all day. Sometimes he won't eat a thing; my husband gets mad and pushes some food into him, which is frequently returned. Everyone is angry or crying. If I prevent the nibbling he gets surly and mean like someone with low blood sugar."

"What would happen if you let him nibble so he at least feels good? Then when your husband comes home, tell him that Kevin had to eat early because of a starvation problem. Then serve Kevin a couple of grapes or a piece of apple and some dried, chipped beef. Children like Kevin overreact to stress and cannot eat if upset; they are so distractible that the actions of others eating prevents them from doing anything about the food on their own plates."

"Or he gets to talking so much he can't eat and it's, 'Shut up and eat, Kevin,' every two minutes."

"Don't fight him; join him. Tell him if he eats the three grapes and the beef, he may tell the family the most exciting thing that happened to him that day. Somehow you have to make mealtime pleasant. After a few months, you may get him to eat like a normal human being."

"Months!"

"You have to decondition him. Anyone who is crying, mean, pokes fun, or says dirty words at the table is politely but firmly moved to another room."

New Wives' Tale: He who eats with children may lose his appetite.

"If you swallow seeds and pits, you will get appendicitis."

"My child has been eating cherries recently, and I don't think he spits out the pits. He has occasional stomach aches. Is he headed for an attack of appendicitis?

I've also heard if you swallow chewing gum, it will cause an obstruction."

"Is your grandmother living with you? I haven't heard these old tales for a long time. Pathologists examine the contents of diseased appendices and find pus and occasionally some dried up fecal matter, but rarely any seeds. Gum goes right through like a glob of vegetable fiber."

"Why the stomach ache?"

"When did you last deworm him?"

"Oh, that again! He sleeps well. Don't wormy children wake up at night?"

"That's true. How about corn, or chocolate, or pork, or milk, or eggs? You might experiment for awhile by leaving them out of his diet."

"How boring."

"Incidentally, appendicitis frequently runs in families. It is supposed to be a constant pain in the lower right side. Food distress is usually about the navel and comes and goes."

New Wives' Tale: If it's bad manners to spit out seeds, you could swallow them.

"Don't swim until one hour after eating."

"On these hot days I can't keep my children out of the neighbor's pool. They eat and swim all day. How much can they eat without getting a cramp and drowning?"

"I would think they would be more likely to get a cramp if they *don't* eat."

"Huh?"

"The cramp is due to the buildup of waste products and the depletion of sugar in the muscles, so it's probably *good* to eat before the exercise. Maybe not a big heavy meal, but frequent small amounts sound sensible."

"Why all this scare talk about swimming and cramps?"

"I don't know. People would be no more likely to have a cramp in the water than a cramp while jogging. Even so, a child should know how to stay afloat using only his arms."

New Wives' Tale: Eat when you want, but learn how to swim.

"Serving beer and wine to children will make them alcoholic when adults."

"My husband thinks it's funny when he lets our three-year-old drink beer. He says it doesn't hurt him, and I say he'll develop a taste for it and grow up to be a sot."

"You both may be right. He may grow up to be a drinker, a nondrinker, or someone in between. I haven't any statistics on this, but my feeling is that children who are nibblers are more likely to find alcohol helpful in adulthood."

"What should I do right now?"

"Like with everything else you do, it is better to offer options and let the child choose the appropriate and most socially acceptable path. If you can somehow indicate that wine and beer are to be used only at mealtime to promote a good appetite and improve dinner table fellowship, then you have done a good job as parents. Drugs and alcohol are used as substitutes when human contacts are unrewarding."

"I have a brother who is—I hate to say it—a drunk. My husband has a couple of odd relatives—loners, he calls them. I may be overreacting."

"Statistics are against you, because there is some familial incidence. But you can beat the statistics—not with an all-out proscription like, 'If you ever touch the stuff, I'll kill you' or 'Bad, evil, sinful people drink; if you do, you'll go straight to hell.' If you make it taboo, you might make it sound exciting. You will do your son a favor if you teach him some form of tolerant acceptance. He's going to be surrounded with dozens of temptations as he grows and moves further away from your surveillance. It is far better for him to discover the pharmacological effects of alcohol in the security of his home than to be hit with its toxic effects in a bar in some strange city when he's eighteen years old."

"Oh, God! My little baby!"

"Don't make it a big imponderable. Don't push it down his throat, but maybe let him sip a little at festive occasions or holidays. Don't make it a big deal. Call it a food; that might remove some of the stigma. Can you get your husband to have his beer with meals?"

"Television sports make him thirsty."

"Giving your son a good self-image by getting him into socially acceptable, fun things that really turn him on will be the best way to help him avoid a few of the evils of life. Don't waste your breath lecturing him. I'm sure you've found that doesn't work with your husband."

"That's for sure."

New Wives' Tale: If you tell your child not to put a bean up his nose, you will have a child with a clogged nostril.

"If you don't eat foods with fats and carbohydrates, you will lose weight."

"My fourteen-year-old daughter is a big, fat slob. Last year you said the plumpness would move around to all the right places on her body and she would look like a female. She's still a teardrop, not an hourglass, and I want something done. Should we see an endocrinologist or a psychiatrist?"

"It would be nice if it were a thyroid problem. Are her palms warm and moist?"

"Yes. Aren't all adolescents like that?"

"Usually. In general that rules out low thyroid function as a cause of obesity. Hypothyroid victims are cold, dry, and sluggish with thickened, waxy skin."

"Sluggish she is, but not the other things."

"Are her periods okay, and how tall is she?"

"She began two years ago and they are now fairly regular. She's about five feet, four inches; she hasn't grown for the last year. Isn't that a sign of low thyroid?"

"Girls grow only an inch or so after their periods begin, but the weight gain should stop."

"She's put on about twelve pounds a year since then. She's up to about 140 pounds and still piling it on. No matter what I say, she just doesn't seem to care how she looks."

"Has she tried a diet or joined one of the groups that help people lose?"

"Both. We both did; I lost and she kept adding on. She thought it was 'stupid.' She seemed to eat less but kept on gaining. She tried the water diet but got tired of going to the bathroom all the time. She tried the lean meat and grapefruit once but it was boring. She thinks if she can't lose forty pounds in a week, the diet is no good."

"What about an exercise program?"

"We did a swimming bit at the local club but she just splashed a little and floated and gained."

"What would happen if you left her alone?"

"I couldn't do that. She'd be up to 200 pounds!"

"You've tried everything else. Maybe she needs a layer of fat to protect her real self inside."

"A buffer zone? You're kidding. She claims she wants to lose."

"Most things we do are a defense against anxiety. It's possible she may know that if she sheds her mantle of fat she will become sexually attractive to some young man. She may be telling you she doesn't want to get involved. It's similar to the situation of a girl going downtown on Saturday with no makeup and her hair up in curlers; she's telling the world that tonight is not the night. Maybe you'd better leave her alone. Girls like this will drop thirty pounds at age sixteen or seventeen with little effort. They're ready."

New Wives' Tale: Inside the fat person is someone you don't even know.

"Athletes should get used to going without water. Drinking fluid during a game will slow you down or give you a stomach cramp."

"My seventeen-year-old is a great athlete but seems completely exhausted in the second half of the game. You just checked his blood before the season and he was not anemic. I know he doesn't smoke or take drugs. Has he got mono? Is he abusing himself—whatever that is?"

"I assume he is motivated."

"Oh, yes! He just lives for sports and he's the leading scorer. This slowdown is just killing him. He becomes very depressed. The coach feels he has great potential and is discouraged to see him so pooped. He wants you to check it out."

"Does he eat and drink okay?"

"Huge amounts. And we give extra protein supplements and all the vitamins. I understand vitamin E is good for energy."

"The only thing that science can prove about vitamin E is that the lack of it makes cattle more prone to miscarriage."

"Great. What do we do?"

"Does he drink some fluid to replace the sweat loss?"

"After he gets home. The coach doesn't want the boys to drink during the game, as it slows them down."

"Does Billy sweat much during the game?"

"He's dripping. He seems to work up a real lather; he really gets involved. He's moving all the time."

"I'll bet that that's the reason. Some coaches don't realize an active player can lose several pounds of water during a fast game on a hot day. It must be replaced. He probably should be taking a salt pill or two between quarters and at the half. I'd better call the coach and explain a few things about fluid balance."

New Wives' Tale: If the body loses water, the liquid must be replaced.

5

"Early to Bed . . ."

Old Wives' Tale: "If a baby sleeps on his stomach, he may smother."

"I'm trying to get my baby to sleep on his side or back, but he just cries and waves his arms about. On his stomach he curls up in the fetal position and sleeps for hours. Can he breathe this way?"

"A normal baby just a few days old can lift his head up. If he spits up something, he has no trouble getting his face out of it. If he is lying on his back and spits up, he may have more trouble getting rid of the material in his throat. Babies sleep face up or face down with no trouble at all. Lying on the stomach allows the windpipe to drain—if it needs to. The mattress should be firm."

"Why do babies smother?"

"Not from the position they sleep in. It's probably from some overwhelming virus, *not* smothering."

"So the stomach is okay?"

"The only problem with the prone position is that these babies often sleep with their buttocks resting on their heels with the toes pointing inward. This can make them quite pigeon-toed unless we watch it. Let him sleep in whatever position is comfortable. We had a baby with so much gas that we had to position him half sitting so he could burp and pass gas more easily."

New Wives' Tale: If a baby is sleeping, he is probably in a comfortable position.

"A child will get a bad cold if he doesn't stay covered."

"My baby never stays under the covers at night. He's like a mole; he tunnels around under the blankets until they are pulled out. Then he comes out on top and I find him in the morning asleep on the wadded blankets. Should I give him some penicillin so he won't get pneumonia?"

"Maybe he's having some exciting, fun-filled dreams. Better not disturb him or confine him."

"Isn't he getting exposed? Should I put him in one of those sleeping bag things with arms so he'll always be covered?"

"Maybe he's uncomfortable under the blanket and is trying to cool off. During sleep the skin capillaries dilate and the body temperature falls, so his skin may seem hot to him. My wife sleeps with one foot and leg outside the covers. It seems odd but she never gets sick."

"How do I know he is comfortable and won't get a chill?"

"Feel down inside his back. If that's warm, he is probably okay. Are his feet warm?"

"Yes. Sometimes they are cold when he has just eaten."

"The nasal capillaries of some people constrict when

they get cold feet. If the room temperature is about 65° to 70° and his feet are warm, he's probably okay. Maybe he doesn't need a blanket; try just some warm socks. Don't strap him in bed though; some babies get all tangled up in those harnesses."

"I don't know what to do. I'd like him covered."

"It may take a few years for him to get used to *your* idea of comfort. We had a restless sleeper in our own family. His turnings in the creaky crib woke us up, so we put the mattress on the floor and let him figure out whatever was suitable. The whole room was his bed; he slept and so did we. He never got a cold until he went to nursery school."

"What about bath time? My mother-in-law heats up the bathroom to 80° or so before she will allow a stitch of clothing to be removed. What does the expert say?"

"A baby's skin is large in proportion to his weight, so he can lose body heat more rapidly than an adult. He might be uncomfortably chilled when his wet skin is exposed to cooler air, but that does not mean he will get a cold."

"What about going outside with wet hair? Doesn't that lead to pneumonia?"

"There are many blood vessels in the scalp, so water vaporizing from this area might have a chilling effect, but this does not lead to a cold or sore throat."

New Wives' Tale: If the skin is cool, warm it up; if it is hot, cool it off.

"Children should sleep with the windows open so they will have fresh air."

"My mother-in-law and I are having an argument about the baby's bedroom. I would like to have the window open an inch or two from the bottom, but she insists on having the window open five or six inches at the top *and* bottom. She says the fresh air is important to lung development. The oxygen will help his brain while he sleeps, and it may prevent tuberculosis."

"I will agree that we all need oxygen, but most houses leak enough around the edges that fresh air gets in and stale air gets out."

"But is it enough? How do I know there is enough oxygen in his room to last all night?"

"Is there a crack under the door?"

"Yes."

"Shut the door and hold a lighted match near the crack and you will notice there is a steady flow of fresh air."

"You're telling me that I don't have to open the window?"

"Yes. If you open the window in the winter, you're just heating up the outdoors and you waste fuel. The only time you should open a window is in a room where a fire is smoldering in the fireplace and carbon monoxide is being produced and the damper is closed. Just leave the door open a crack. Tell grandmother that tuberculosis comes from people who have tuberculosis."

New Wives' Tale: Opening the bedroom window makes the room cold.

"To get a baby to sleep through the night, give him solids."

"My baby is three weeks old, and I'd like him to sleep through the night. What's the best way to get him to do it?"

"Don't be too discouraged if nothing works except time. Most people try rice cereal mixed with a little warm formula. The problem is that it takes about twenty minutes to scoop it in and poke it down his gullet. After all this work and frustration you will be lucky if he sleeps twenty minutes longer. It hardly seems worth it."

"I'd like to try. All my friends gave solids early."

"Some recent research suggests that those babies given solids early are more likely to be obese adults. Allergists warn us that early solid food feedings may increase the likelihood of the development of food allergies."

"Come off it! I want some sleep."

"How tall are you?"

"Five feet six; my husband is six feet. Why?"

"You are taller than average, so your baby may not be able to crowd enough calories down during the day to fuel his nighttime growth. Babies of short parents sleep through the night right away."

"Doesn't cereal have a lot of calories?"

"Yes. Milk has twenty calories per ounce, and an ounce of dry cereal has a hundred calories; so it *should* do something. Some claim that a little strained meat at night makes the baby last all night. However, the extra salt and minerals are thought to be a burden on the kidneys."

"Well, let me try it anyway."

"Sure. Don't overdo it and don't fight him It's got to be fun for both of you."

"I'll smile as I poke it at him."

"Remember the only real reason that solids are introduced early in the first year is to preclude the common milk anemia that follows an exclusively milk diet."

"Okay, I get the message. How do I prevent that?"

"Many milks are now iron fortified. Try one. I have

the feeling that if Mother Nature wanted babies to have solids early, teeth would have been provided. Teeth usually come at about six to eight months of age. This should be the clue that it's time for solids."

New Wives' Tale: Babies sleep through the night when they are ready.

"A child who screams at night is insecure."

"My three-year-old was a good sleeper until she began nursery school. They must be pushing her to conform or scaring her. She's been at the school for two months now, and in the last few nights she has been screaming out at night. She tears up the bed as if wrestling with something and grinds her teeth as if tense. She is crabby and snarly during the day. The teacher says she seems happy in school. Maybe she controls her feelings there only to take them out on me at home. Could you phone the teacher and find out what they're doing to her to make her unhappy and insecure? I'd take her out of the school if we hadn't paid for the whole year. Some of the other mothers report the same problem with their children."

"I've usually felt that an insecure child was afraid to go to bed. Does she mind going to bed and to sleep?"

"No problem. She had that sleep resistance thing at age two, but that's okay now. She does seem frightened when she wakes up, as if she'd had a bad dream. She would like to come into our bed but my husband says 'no' to that."

"I think he's right. I would feel it humane to reassure her when she does awaken, but don't start that terrible habit of allowing her to sleep with you."

"Is it a phase? Should we give her a sleeping pill?"

"Sleeping medicine usually excites a child at this age. Something physical awakens children at night."

"You mean an earache or a toothache?"

"Right; gas or a charley horse muscle cramp. Do you know the most common cause of night wakefulness in children?"

"Hunger?"

"Pinworms!"

"Oh, dear. I should have known. You have a reputation for believing everything is due to worms."

"I've been talking to parents on the phone for more than twenty years and almost every day someone calls about these ubiquitous pests. You don't even have to look for them; all the symptoms are there. The only thing you didn't say is that she has an itchy anus. Does she?"

"Well, she does tug at her underwear as if it's too tight."

"I may be wrong, but we have to start someplace. Before you blame the school, let's blame the worms she got from those friends of hers who have the symptoms. I'll call a prescription in to the druggist. In three nights she should sleep soundly again, and we can assume we made the right diagnosis. Then tell the other mothers what you did, so they may do the same thing before she gets them back again."

"Ugh! Must I really? How embarrassing."

"It just means she socializes well. If this doesn't work, a bladder infection might be responsible. I missed a duodenal ulcer in a child because I didn't think of it; the pain was worse at night because her stomach was empty and the acid was burning a hole in her intestine. Another child had a bone disease that was more painful at night. But pinworms are really at the top of the list."

New Wives' Tale: A child who screams out at night is in pain.

"Children who wet the bed are insecure."

"My boy is six years old and still wets the bed. I've heard that this means he is insecure, or nervous, or unhappy. He does laugh and cry easily and talks too much and too loudly, but school is okay and he has a couple of friends. I try to show love, but I probably make a terrible face when I go into his room and get a whiff of the awful urine smell. What can I do?"

"Is his daytime control okay?"

"Yes. When he has to go, he has to go *right then,* but usually he can wait three or four hours between times."

"Sounds okay. We've tested his urine here sometime in the last year or so. Let me ask you something: did his father have the same trouble?"

"He did mutter something about wetting a couple of times as a child."

"Ask your mother-in-law. She may give you a different idea. We have found a definite familial tendency with enuresis—but don't make your husband feel guilty."

"Is the fact that he's going into first grade responsible?"

"Stress can make it worse. Sometimes children work so hard during the day that they sleep more soundly at night and don't get the message from the full bladder. The bladder has no social consciousness; it really doesn't care where it empties."

"I try not to scold him."

"Right. You can't scold the bladder for doing its thing. The brain and nervous system control-mechanisms are so busy with dreams that the message from the bladder can't get through to awaken the cortex and get him to the bathroom."

"Then he's not insecure or nervous?"

"He may get that way because bed-wetting boys often get a bad self-image. You have to try to ignore this problem and support his flagging ego in other areas—sports, maybe."

"Okay, but isn't there anything we can do?"

"There is a medicine that will keep him from sleeping too soundly and increase the tone of the sphincter muscle that holds the urine in place."

"Call it in to the druggist, quick!"

"Okay, but you might try the allergy approach also. A few children wet because of an allergy to milk or citrus or chocolate. Try it; you'll know in just a day or so."

"How about those machines that ring a bell when urine closes the electric circuit?"

"Sometimes they work in the older boy who might be more motivated. Usually the family awakens while the child sleeps right on through."

"What a drag!"

"Hyperactive children are more likely to wet, probably because of a genetic defect in the neurochemical connections in the lower part of the brain. Take heart; he'll outgrow it."

"I suppose if my husband had told me he had a bad gene before we were married, I would have married him anyway."

New Wives' Tale: Children who wet the bed may **become** ***insecure.***

"A growing child needs nine to ten hours' sleep."

"We have a wild, flighty child who doesn't seem to fit into our household pattern. Take bedtime, for instance: he won't go to bed when we ask, so we get tough and soon we are all screaming at each other. This just stimulates him and he is awake for hours. Even when he goes to bed on time, he may not fall asleep until after our bedtime at 11:00 P.M. He's not getting enough sleep, is he?"

"Can he get up in the morning?"

"Oh, yes. He's up before we are sometimes and has breakfast ready. His idea of breakfast is a dozen eggs with a few shells cooked without butter over the high burner, Cheerios, strawberry jam, and milk over everything. Where does he get the energy?"

"His early awakening would suggest to me that he's getting enough sleep. His body may know more than we do. Maybe you ought to let him decide when he should go to sleep. You can't force that on him."

"Apparently. But he has to go to bed before he can go to sleep."

"True. You can order *that.* Why don't you get him to bed at 8:00 or 9:00 P.M. and allow him to have a bedside light on. Tell him he may read or play a quiet game, and you will get mad only if he is noisy or comes out and bothers the family."

"Sounds like we're letting him get away with something."

"No, you're just accepting a fact of life, like the color of his eyes. When you go to bed, tiptoe in and turn off the light and kiss him goodnight—unless that wakes him up. One mother told me that when she tried this technique, the boy went to sleep earlier and more easily, probably because he wasn't upset with the usual angry argument."

New Wives' Tale: Don't fight the natural rhythm of the body; remember, the elbow bends only one way.

6

Ounces of Prevention, Pounds of Cure

Old Wives' Tale: "Cold and dampness cause colds."

"We came to Oregon a few months ago and have had colds and coughs constantly. Shall we move back to California or take vitamin C? This dampness is going to kill us."

"Well, we are trying to keep soreheads out of the state, but I protest the implication that our state is unhealthy. You know, we turn on the vaporizers when the air is dry. People in Arizona report a bad form of croup in their dry weather when the night temperature drops from 100° down to 40°."

"If it's so great here, why are we sick so much?"

"If you could maintain the temperature at 65° to 70°, keep the humidity at about 50 percent, and eliminate the various viruses that cause colds, you'd have it made."

"Most people can't do that and they don't get sick."

"The unknown quantity is individual susceptibility, which is somehow related to allergies. You've got to clean the furnace, eliminate house dust, keep the dog outside, put some kind of plastic over the dirt under the house to control mold, or move to another house."

New Wives' Tale: Colds are due to viruses, but susceptibility is due to allergies.

"If you have an allergy, get an allergist to do some skin tests."

"I'm sick and tired of my child picking his nose all the time. I treated him for worms, but he still does it. What's next?"

"Sounds like an allergy. Is it year-round?"

"Yes, but worse now in the early summer. Should we see an allergist?"

"Maybe. Some allergies are so multiple and so occult that the allergist is essential. But you can have the fun of the detective work and get some credit for the control by trying a few things. Is he a blue-eyed blond?"

"Yes. What does that have to do with it?"

"We were taught in medical school that the freckle-faced redhead is the allergy-prone person, but the blue-eyed blond is more likely to have the inherited allergic tendencies. It's some genetic problem."

"My husband and I are fair. He sneezes when he mows the lawn, and I have to hire a cleaning lady because I get asthma when I vacuum the house."

"That's a clue. Didn't your son have to drink soy bean milk as an infant?"

"Yes, but he's okay now on cow's milk."

"Maybe he isn't. Does he have circles under his eyes? Does he make that zonking sound like he's trying to clear the phlegm from the back of his nose?"

"Doesn't everybody?"

'Well, not all the time. If you look hard enough you'll find some allergy to *something* in everybody. The idea is to remove the worst offenders from the environment and the diet and see if the child is more comfortable. We already know that he has been allergic to milk—and may still be. Why don't you start with the elimination of milk, ice cream, and cottage cheese and see if the zonking is at least less? The nose-picking is usually a sign of an inhalation allergy, like your house dust or your husband's grass. How many colds a year does he have?"

"A year? It's more like one or two a month. I give him vitamin C, but it hasn't helped."

"Frequent colds and respiratory infections mean allergy. Many people blame our rainy weather as the cause of their colds. Susceptibility is increased by an allergy. A dirt basement frequently grows mold which serves as an allergen. If any part of your house is placed over open dirt, cover that dirt with a big sheet of plastic. If that doesn't work, you might consider moving. Some people buy an electronic precipitator, which removes pollen, mold, and dust from the air—and is tax deductible."

"So is an allergist."

"He's going to make you change the environment, too. If you do some of these simple things, maybe you won't need the allergist. Maybe you're telling me you would like to see him. Is he a symbol?"

"No, it's just that some of my friends have been the allergy route and are so much better now."

"It's no big mystery. We ordinary doctors have learned a few things also. Much of allergy is common sense detective work. I forgot to ask: is the mucus from his nose green, yellow, or clear?"

"There are always some crusty goobers there, and when it does run it's a chartreuse color. Why?"

"Aha! That's a secondary infection. Colored stuff means a germ has gotten in on top of the allergy. Let me give him three or four shots of a vaccine containing a mixture of the usual bacteria found in everyone's nose. These shots of this dead bacteria are supposed to teach him how to fight off his infections better. If the mucus that remains is clear, and he sneezes and rubs his nose, then he is inhaling some irritant. If it's clear and he just zonks, then the trouble is more likely diet—usually milk."

New Wives' Tale: If you are allergic to something, remove it.

"Stuff a cold and starve a fever."

"My child has a cold and a fever; am I supposed to feed him or starve him?"

"Neither. Just give him a lot of fluids. I don't know where that old saying came from. I suppose it comes from the fact that many people vomit when they have a fever. Aspirin and water are easier to clean up."

New Wives' Tale: If your child is sick, make him comfortable.

"If a patient is having a chill, wrap him up in a blanket."

Phone call, 8:00 P.M.: "Our three-year-old felt dumpy this afternoon after play. I thought he was just tired, so I fed him a light supper which he barely ate. He was so drowsy he almost fell into the Jello. We put him to bed and he went right to sleep. Just now he woke up and threw up all over the bed. Now he has a chill so we've wrapped him up in a blanket. Has he got malaria or just the flu?"

"Take him out of the blanket and get him in a hot bath."

Pause. "A *hot* bath?"

"Yes. The chill means his fever is going up and you must move his body heat to the skin surface so he can radiate the heat into the air."

Second pause. "A *hot* bath?"

"A hot bath. Real hot water is only 96° or so, which is cooler than his inside temperature. His skin is cool to the touch if he is having a chill, so it cannot dissipate the heat that his shaking muscles are generating."

"A hot bath."

"You have to make the skin red in the bath and then let the water evaporate from his skin. The vaporization of the water is the mechanism by which the hot blood in the skin is cooled. Like throwing water on a hot stove—it doesn't matter if the water is hot or cold; the stove is cooled when the water is changed to steam. It also cleans the patient if I have to examine him," I say, trying to interject a little cheer into a frightening experience.

"A hot bath."

"Get his skin good and red; then if you like you may put him naked on a towel on the bed and sponge his body back and forth with a wet washcloth. His skin has to be hot and red or the water won't evaporate. When you sponge him use warm water; cold is too uncomfortable. Don't use alcohol; it is very cooling but some children inhale too much of the fumes and get toxic."

"Well, you're the doctor."

"Try to get some aspirin in him. Take his temperature now. Give him the aspirin (one grain for each ten pounds of body weight), then give him the hot bath for twenty minutes. Then sponge him for twenty minutes, then put him in light pajamas and cover him with only a sheet. In an hour and a half from now his temperature should be down one or two degrees and he should be sleeping reasonably comfortably. You must call me back by 10:00 P.M. if he is no better. If he's cooler, that suggests it is the flu or some crud that is going around. If he is not better, I should see him tonight to rule out pneumonia, kidney infection, or something serious."

New Wives' Tale: If the body is cold to the touch, warm it up. If it is hot, cool it down.

"A child with measles should be kept in a dark room."

"We somehow forgot to get the measles shot for our son and now he has the cough, red eyes, and fever, and is breaking out. He wants to watch his favorite TV show. Doesn't the light wreck his eyes?"

"His eyes are sensitive to light because they are so inflamed, but the light itself will not damage the eyes. Any damage might come from the virus in the nervous system which might invade some critical brain cells."

"Really?"

"The *content* of the TV program is the thing to worry about."

New Wives' Tale: The only light to worry about is the strong rays from direct viewing of the sun.

"Take flu shots (or vitamin C or E) to avoid the flu."

"My whole family had the flu two or three times last year. The symptoms were fever, aching eyeballs, strangley cough that lasted for three weeks, and weakness. We've been taking vitamin C for some time and have been well, but we'd like the flu shot, too."

"Really, the only way to avoid the flu is to stay locked

up in the attic for the winter and receive no visitors. But then the bug would come in on some Christmas card and get you."

"Will you give us the flu shot, or do we go to another doctor, or get them free at work?"

"Okay, okay, I'll give them. But remember, there is no guarantee. It's hard to predict which strain is going to be the 'virus that's going around' because it's a different virus every year."

"The standard disclaimer, eh?"

"If I give you all the shot and you get the flu, you'll blame me. Actually, it sounds as if you are ahead of the flu game. You've *had* all of the ones going around, so you should be immune for a year or so. Whatever you do will get the credit. I took Dr. Jarvis's vinegar and honey routine for a year or so. I ran out of vinegar and lost faith in the treatment. Then I came down with the worst cold I've ever had."

New Wives' Tale: Do something safe and practical for your health, but be sure you have faith in it.

"A child who picks his nose has worms."

"Would you call in some more worm medicine? Carolyn is picking her nose."

"Does she do anything else?"

"Yes, she sits on cold cement and eats candy a lot."

"No, I mean, does she have stomach aches and night wakefulness?"

"Don't all kids have those things?"

"Really, now. Pinworms are busy at night, usually one to four hours after the child goes to sleep. If she has worms she's supposed to cry out at night, scratch her anal area, and maybe have a nightmare."

"She does those things, too. But where does she keep getting them? From the candy or the cement?"

"If she has wormy friends, she will get them. Pinworm infestation is a social disease of children. We adults have ours; they have theirs. Nose-picking is a sign of hay fever; she is inhaling some dander or pollen that makes her nose itch. Children with hay fever are more susceptible to pinworm infestation because they have their hands near their mouths more. Thumbsuckers and nailbiters frequently get worms. Their hands carry the pinworm eggs to their mouths."

New Wives' Tale: Children frequently have worms; it means they have friends.

"To stop a nosebleed, put a cold knife on the back of the neck."

"My eight-year-old boy has bloody noses all the time. I've heard this means rheumatic fever or some awful blood disease."

"We can easily check out those diseases with a few simple blood tests. How do you stop the bleeding?"

"I get him to blow his nose to get rid of the clots and have him lie down with something cold on his neck, like ice or a cold knife. They finally stop, but it takes so long. And in two days he has another one."

"There's an old truism: bleeding always stops. But what a waste! One could get anemic from chronic blood loss. When you want to stop the flow of water in the garden hose, you step on it. Blood is circulated in tubes; you must squash the vessels flat to stop the bleeding. Most noses bleed from the capillary bed in the first one-half to one inch of the septum, so the idea is to pinch the nose tight at the tip—not the bridge. You have to hold it snug for about ten to fifteen minutes; the clotting mechanisms take about that long to plug up the capillaries. It helps to wet a piece of cotton or tissue, wad it up so it just fits in the nostril, shove it in, and like a tampon it gives something to squeeze on. It is also helpful to have the patient sit up or even lean forward. This maneuver prevents the blood from running back down the throat and nauseating him; also you can tell when the bleeding stops. Pinch ten minutes, wait ten minutes, then slowly pull the cotton out. This leaves a clear open space and very little clot."

"You mean I have to sit on this kid all that time? I can't even get him to sit still long enough to comb his hair!"

"Well, yes. You're bigger than he is. Maybe you can get him to pinch it tight himself. Sometimes it hurts less to pinch one's own nose. He has to learn to do it. After the bleeding stops, teach him to poke a small dab of an antibiotic ointment up his nose. This lubricates the area."

"Yeah. Sure."

"Most erosions take about seven days to heal. So if it bleeds again within the week, add another seven days to the healing process. Someday soon come in and I'll touch up the area with some silver nitrate. This scars down the capillaries and may stop future leaks."

"Sure."

"I heard of a man who had tried everything for nosebleed and found the best, for him, was to put ice on his testicles."

"Wonderful."

New Wives' Tale: If the nose is bleeding, do something about the nose.

"If you get a burn, put raw onion, lard, or butter on it."

"I've heard of the benefits of onions, but I didn't have a chance to try it until a few days ago. I was cooking some hamburgers when two globs of grease came flying out and landed on my forearm. Because the raw sliced onion was handy, I tried a controlled experiment: I held a piece of onion on one of the burns and left the other one open to the air. Now, four days later, the onion-treated burn is brownish and healing and the untreated one is red and raw. I thought you'd like to know; maybe you could write it up in a medical journal."

"Well, let me tell you what science has been doing; you're not the only one running experiments. They asked some prisoners to cooperate and promised them early parole if they would. These men were burned equally on both sides of their abdomen. One side was treated with a bland ointment and the other was covered with a layer of wet gauze on top of which was chopped ice. This remained for two to four hours. Complete healing of the second-degree burn was accomplished on the ice side in about one-half the time that it took for the untreated side."

"Don't you like onions?"

"I didn't say that. I said ice or ice water—not cold water—is best for the usual second-degree or small, possibly third-degree burn. Plunge a hand or foot in a bucket of ice water; or a little plastic bag with ice water can be slipped over a hand and wrapped with a towel. It must be left on for one to three hours. This apparently prevents the poisons made by the burned tissue from causing further damage to the next layer of skin underneath. It also eases the pain."

"Why do onions work?"

"Science will find the answer. The onion industry is sponsoring research in this. Onion juice makes a great cough syrup. The core of a boiled onion stuck in the ear hole usually stops an earache. But ice is the best thing for burns."

New Wives' Tale: If a part of the body is hot, cool it off.

"Put mud or fresh cow manure on a bee sting."

"We visited Grandma on the farm and our six-year-old was attacked by yellow jackets. His leg was stung in several places. Grandma got a sheet and followed a cow around until she got some fresh manure. She packed his leg in this for several hours and the next day you could barely find the bites. I thought you'd like to know this so you could tell other patients or tell the A.M.A. or somebody."

"Say that once more."

She does.

"I've heard of things like that, but not in school. The toxin that bees inject causes a release of histamine which causes the big, red, itchy swelling. We recommend an antihistamine immediately following the bite; it would be better before, if possible."

New Wives' Tale: Use an antihistamine for bee stings if fresh cow manure is not available.

"Don't touch a person with poison ivy or poison oak, or you will get it."

"My six-year-old was exploring in the nearby woods yesterday, and today he has a wild, red, blistery, burning, itchy rash. I'm afraid to pat any lotion on him because I might get it; I'm very susceptible."

"Did you wash the clothes he was wearing?"

"Yes, I knew about that. And he had a bath, but the rash continues to spread. I've got a couple of spots on my hands and forearms already."

"That's probably from the poisonous residue in the clothing, or it's in his dog's fur and you touched that. They did some research on poison ivy and found if the skin is bathed within thirty minutes of contact, the rash is less likely to develop. After that the allergic reaction has already begun and bathing is not effective. You are no more likely to get a rash by touching his skin than you would get a burn by touching a person with a sunburn."

"Why does it spread, then?"

"Some areas take longer to break out than others. But it's five days getting worse and five days getting better. If he can't sleep because of the discomfort, come in and we'll give him a cortisone shot. I remember seeing a case of poison oak in a baby ten months old who had crawled over the living room rug where his father had walked after trampling in the stuff while fishing."

New Wives' Tale: Poison ivy and poison oak are not contagious through personal contact.

"If your toes, fingers, nose, or ears are frostbitten, rub them with snow."

"We were playing out in the snow and cold and must not have noticed our feet icing up. We rubbed them with snow. Now the skin of some of the toes is falling off like that of a burn. What do we do now?"

I sigh, a little discouraged. "I thought everyone knew now that hot water is the thing to use for frostbite, but I suppose you were a long way from home." Not wanting to antagonize the patient, I give him an excuse to use.

"Yeah. Right. But wouldn't that hurt to plunge them in hot water?"

"Not as much as what you are suffering now or might have if you had gotten gangrene." Doctors like to use the scare approach; it sometimes works. "Incidentally, clean dry socks are a good way to insulate the feet from cold. As soon as they get dirty and/or sweat-soaked, they're no longer able to hold a thin layer of dead air as a buffer zone."

"Okay."

Here comes the lecture. "The rapid immersion of the frostbitten skin into hot water (100° to 105°) rapidly serves to melt the ice crystals inside the cells. If the cell freezes, its wall ruptures, as the milk bottle cap rises when the milk freezes. Rubbing adds insult to the already injured tissues. One mountain climber told me they nestled their cold toes in each others' armpits for warmth."

"Okay, okay."

New Wives' Tale: If the body is cold, warm it up.

"Use boric acid solution for irritated or infected eyes."

"My baby has sticky, yellow matter in his eyes. How often should I be putting the boric acid solution in his eyes?"

"I'm sorry to have to tell you this, but you shouldn't be using boric acid. Thirty years ago it was about the only thing, along with ammoniated mercury, that was available for eye infections and conjunctivitis."

"What's the matter with it? Grandmother says it's really the best thing for eyes. She used to use it in the diaper rinse to get rid of the ammonia, too."

"A few years ago some deaths were reported from

its use in diapers; the acid was absorbed through open skin sores and caused an overwhelming acidosis. Occasionally boric acid has been mistakenly used as salt or sugar. It's a severe poison."

"What if I'm careful?"

"We have an axiom: If there is a child and a poison in the same house, they will find each other. Get rid of it. There is no reason to have it. The druggist shouldn't have sold it to you. He shouldn't even stock it."

"Okay, okay. What do I use?"

"I'll call in a prescription for some antibiotic ointment."

"Penicillin?"

"No. It's best not to use the same antibiotic in the eye or on the skin that may be used internally. Sensitivity is easily developed this way."

New Wives' Tale: For infected eyes use a medicine that kills just the bacteria, not the patient.

"To get rid of warts: pray, bury a washcloth, have grandmother buy them, rub them with potato, iodine, swamp water, and so on."

"My child has some ugly warts on her hands and we've tried everything. Can science help?"

"Yes. Some of the things we do make them go away before they would disappear spontaneously. If we treat them at the moment of involution, we may be credited with a cure. Today's treatment is a drop of an extract of June bugs. It has a vesicant or blister-making property, and separates the wart from underlying normal skin. This material, incidentally, has been used as an aphrodisiac. So perhaps it gets the wart so excited it falls off."

"Does it hurt?"

"On the wart? The application doesn't, but sometimes the blister becomes painful until it breaks. Along with the local treatment I try some self-hypnosis. I make the patient say, 'The wart is going away.' But they must not smile."

"You're kidding."

"No. We know that there is some magic to positive thinking. Medicine, Christian Science, acupuncture, chiropractic, faith healing—we all use it to some extent. There is a term called 'placebo effect.' Many patients get well if the doctor looks them in the eye and tells them to get well. My headaches go away even before the aspirin reaches my stomach because I have faith in aspirin."

"What do you charge?"

"Seven dollars, but that includes return visits until it's gone."

"Grandmother's cheaper."

"But slower. Is your daughter getting a bad self-image from the warts?"

"You and that self-image again."

"Okay, but some people still believe warts come from playing with yourself. We now know they are due to a virus."

"I'll come in tomorrow."

New Wives' Tale: Some problems may disappear with faith, but science can make faith more efficient.

"A broken rib should be taped."

"Our son fell off his bike yesterday, and his chest must have hit the curb or something because it hurts him to breathe."

"Sounds like he broke a rib."

"Oh, dear. Should I get an X ray or something?"

"If he seems all right otherwise and isn't coughing up blood, and you don't need X rays for insurance purposes, you can let it go. Broken ribs are painful for a week or so, but heal easily."

"Don't you tape the chest?"

"That was standard until recently. But a few patients developed pneumonia because the taping restricted deep breathing."

"What about the pain?"

"Aspirin is usually not enough. I'll call in a prescription for codeine to your druggist. Give it to your son for a few days. If he gets worse after tomorrow, call back and I'll examine him and maybe get some X rays."

New Wives' Tale: Don't start overtreating a problem before you have to.

"If you hit your head, you'd better get an X ray."

"My baby just fell off the Bathinette. I just turned around for a second to get a diaper and he flipped over!"

"Easy. What's he doing now?"

"He screamed and got all red. Now he's quiet and pale. Shall I take him to the hospital?"

"Hold it. Let's just talk for a while and see what he does for the next few minutes. While he was crying did he seem to move everything?"

"Oh, yes. He was kicking his legs and flailing his arms around wildly."

"It's not a perfect rule, but your description suggests there are no big bones broken."

"I'm worried about his head. What if he's cracked his skull?"

"It's possible, but the skull bone is not as important as the brain inside. Any injury to the brain will make it swell up. It's called concussion, which may sound scary, but it goes away. It's the same type of swelling that you get in a muscle after a blow. But when the brain swells inside the skull, headache, vomiting, and drowsiness occur. These symptoms take six to twelve hours to develop and anywhere up to several days to subside. How does he seem now?"

"He's pale and quiet. I'm frightened."

"Pinch his heel and see how he responds."

"He grimaces and pulls his foot away from me."

"Good. He's responding. This means a message is getting up to his brain and back down again to the leg muscles. He's in a deep sleep."

"Shouldn't I keep him awake?"

"No. He needs the rest to repair the injury. But rouse him every twenty minutes by pinching his heel or poking him. You want to see how deeply he is asleep and how easily rousable he is."

"Shouldn't a nurse in the hospital be watching him?"

"If he gets more difficult to rouse, she may be able to help us by monitoring pulse and blood pressure. But you're his mother and you will be better able to detect personality changes or subtle derangements of sleep, activity, and appetite. Why don't you see how he gets along for the next few hours? Shall I call you in four hours?"

"I think I feel better."

New Wives' Tale: If you hit your head, take a nap.

"Every puncture wound needs a tetanus shot."

"My nine-year-old boy was playing in an abandoned house a little while ago and stepped on an old rusty nail. I thought I'd better call to say we were rushing over to the hospital emergency room to get a tetanus booster so he won't get lockjaw."

"I'm glad you called. I may be able to save you a little time and money. Some recent research has indicated that we are giving too many tetanus booster shots. The tetanus shot has indeed saved many lives; I understand that of all the thousands of soldiers wounded in World War II, only a handful died of tetanus, and some in this group may not have been properly immunized."

"Can you talk faster? We're about to leave."

"Wait a minute. You pressed my tetanus button and you might as well hear the whole commerical. He got his baby shots, didn't he?"

"Yes, but that was nine years ago. Don't you remember how he screamed?"

"Sorry, I'd almost forgotten. We usually give a booster at age two years and again at age five, just before kindergarten."

"Well, we've always brought him in to you and assumed you would give him what he needed."

"Right. And that's the point. The research suggests that after those initial three DPT (diphtheria-pertussis-tetanus) shots the body will be protected against a tetanus invasion for up to thirty years."

"Shouldn't we get one to make sure?"

"Some people get quite ill with these shots, so some compromise is worthwhile. We now say if the baby DPT series has been given along with the two- and five-year-old boosters, then a routine DT booster is necessary only every ten years (pertussis omitted after age five). If more than five years have gone by or the wound is very contaminated—like a barnyard manure fork puncture—then a booster is suggested."

"You're telling me we can forget it?"

"Yes. Call the office tomorrow and find out for sure if a booster was given to him at age five. If it's over five years since the last booster, come to the office for it either tomorrow or the next day."

"But if he needs a booster, shouldn't he get it now?"

"Tetanus takes a while to develop. We have a couple of days to get the booster into him to stir up his immune defense system. It's also cheaper to come to the office than to the emergency room. They may give only the tetanus, anyway. If we give a booster we might as well protect him against diphtheria also."

"My husband couldn't wait. They just drove off to the emergency room."

New Wives' Tale: Not every emergency is an emergency.

"Wonder drugs have licked everything."

"My child had a fever yesterday and complained of a sore throat. We had some leftover penicillin so we gave him three tablets. His fever is still up, he has a barking cough, and his torso is all broken out. Is this scarlet fever? Your book says a fever, sore throat, and rash could be a strep infection. Isn't penicillin good for strep?"

"Sorry, but you shouldn't start treating before you establish the diagnosis. Naughty, naughty. About ten diseases can give that combination of sore throat, fever, and rash."

"How about scarlet fever? Don't you treat that right away?"

"Yes, but because scarlet fever is a strep, it always

responds to penicillin. He'd be almost well today from the penicillin you gave him. But his fever is still up, so that rules out a strep. Now we have to figure out if the rash is due to a penicillin allergy or to the virus in his bloodstream dilating his blood vessels."

"How do we treat him now? He's still sick."

"Most infections in children are due to viruses, and we have no treatment for them yet. The barking cough tends to rule out a strep and suggests influenza, which is a virus. Antibiotics given during a virus infection can allow a resistant germ to develop."

"I thought modern medicine had solved all this."

"The biochemists and engineers have done more for health than the doctors have. The new vaccines have eliminated some bad infections, and sewage treatment has cut down on intestinal infections, but viruses are still the big troublemakers."

"Back to aspirin and fluid and call tomorrow, eh?"

"That's about it. Sorry."

New Wives' Tale: Wonder drugs should be used for diseases that wonder drugs are used for.

7

School Days

Old Wives' Tale: "The IQ test measures a child's intelligence so that he can be placed in school more accurately."

"We just had a school conference with the teacher, the principal, and the school psychologist. They did some testing on John, our eight-year-old boy, because he hasn't been progressing very well. They won't tell me everything about the test. They say his IQ is average but won't give me a number. Will you find out for me?"

"Sure. I can request a copy of the report that the psychologist makes, but none of us is supposed to give you a number like 85 or 100 or 105, whatever it is. It's a good general rule. If someone knows the IQ number is low, the person so pegged may be treated as if it were low, and he may 'become' dull due to lack of stimulation."

"What do you mean?"

"I remember a psychological study in which the teacher was given the IQ numbers for her class and asked to verify the test. After a couple of months the teacher reported to the psychologist that it was fairly accurate: most of the 80–90 IQ children seemed slow and most of the 110–120 IQ children seemed bright. The psychologist admitted that he gave the teacher the children's locker numbers (80–120). The teacher knew the low ones were slow so she treated them that way and they responded correspondingly. She found the higher numbered children were bright and responsive because she treated them as if they were. The IQ score can vary daily within ten points, depending on the approach of the psychologist, the amount of sleep the child had, or whether he had breakfast or not. So the testers are loath to tell parents the exact number in case they are wrong or in case the parents might treat the child differently. So what does the school want to do with your son?"

"Although his IQ is average, they think he's not working up to his potential and repeating the grade might be best to 'consolidate' his education. Won't he be discouraged?"

"Only for a while. He might feel he is the top dog in the new class and become a happy winner. Did they say there was a spread in performance and verbal test scores?"

"They did say something about that. What does it mean?"

"It *suggests* that there is a minor dysfunction of the nervous system. It can mean he's hyperactive."

"Not *that* again. What do we do?"

"They're the educators. You are well advised to follow their suggestion and hold him back. I've seen the unfortunate result of not cooperating with the school. Sometimes teachers and administrators take it out on the child and pressure him into a failure situation to indicate that the parents were wrong. So play their game. They may be right."

New Wives' Tale: The IQ test measures whatever the IQ test is supposed to measure.

"Never hold a child back; you may hurt his self image."

"The teacher says my boy is immature and should repeat the first grade. I'm so upset; he tries so hard. I think if he flunks first grade it will kill him!"

"She may be right. Is he really at the bottom of the class?"

"If he isn't, then he's at the top of those who are doing poorly."

"Does she think he has the potential?"

"She thinks he's got the wherewithal but can't seem to use it because he won't settle down. He is noisy, busy, can't finish his work, does messy work, and bothers the others."

"He sounds somewhat hyperactive."

"If you want him on some medicine, I'd just as soon not go that route. He's got to learn to control his impulses some time."

"Hyperactivity is a nonspecific reaction to stress. We have to find out if he cannot cope because of low IQ, allergy, anemia, defective vision or hearing, or some nervous system fault like dyslexia."

"Wow! What do we do?"

"Let me check out the common physical reasons and hope it's some easily correctable thing like vision. If not, a psychological test may peg his IQ. Some bright children cannot settle down because of boredom. I have a source person that I use to test for reading disability.

Just in the last ten years we have found we can do a lot for these children who don't fit the mold. Our main job is to correct correctable problems so the child will be comfortable in his class. Medicine may be necessary if all these systems are functioning adequately but we find he is mainly an overreacting, touchy boy."

"We think he is sensitive."

"Thank you. That really is a better word. You know, Winston Churchill was like this. They threw him out of school and his mother took over his education. He went on to write a history of World War II and of the English-speaking people—among other things. If he had stayed in school, we might be goose-stepping today."

"What if everything checks out okay?"

"Holding him back a grade—call it repeating first grade—is a wiser thing to do now than risking another year of failure. Next year he could be at the top of the first-grade class. These sensitive people need to feel successful. This more than compensates for the temporary depression associated with being held back."

New Wives' Tale: Holding a child back may be the best thing that could happen to him.

"Teach with the aid of a hickory stick."

"You probably remember my son. He's the one who kicked you when you were giving him his checkup before the first grade. Well, he's in the first grade now, but he may soon be out again, because he did the same thing to his teacher."

"What happened?"

"He was out of his seat for the umpteenth time, and the teacher tried to force him to sit still and finish a spelling lesson. He didn't like this, so he kicked her shin.

She got mad and spanked him. The principal called and said maybe he'd better stay home until we teach him self-control. I'm so embarrassed. I've been crying all day."

"Did he give you any choices? Not even half days?"

"He said they couldn't make any exceptions. Besides he probably hates school now. Recess and lunch are the only reasons he goes."

"Tell me about his kindergarten days."

"It was okay because they offered a variety of things: paint a little, march a little, sing a little—nothing that required much of an attention span. He wandered about during story time, but the teacher ignored him. Now he has to sit still and learn."

"Sounds like he's learning to hate school. Do you think his potential is up to first grade? Should he go back to kindergarten?"

"He writes his name, reads a few words, draws a man complete with ten fingers and a neck, and knows the alphabet. I'm afraid he would be bored to death."

"School must be a joy. Learning has to be fun. It's too bad the school budget can't afford extra teaching help for these hyperactive children so that they could be in smaller classes and each child could work on a contract basis."

"What's that?"

"He signs a contract stating that he will do so many math problems and read so many pages before the week is out. He is given choices: do the work in class, in the library, or at home. He competes with himself and is not left at the bottom of the class pecking order.

"Would spanking help teach him to sit still?"

"I doubt that it would work for more than a day or two. He might feel that you're against him also. We know he can see, can hear, and has enough brains. The school should learn to join him, not fight him. If they punish him, they'll teach him hate. Then when he throws a rock through the school window, they'll wonder why."

"What do we do?"

"There is a medicine that will control his hyperactivity. If he is better, the school will be able to compliment his good attitude and completed work. He will begin to think school is fun. It breaks the vicious cycle. Sometimes the teacher can bend a few rules for these children and let them work in the library where there are fewer distractions. I know a teacher who recognizes an active child's need to move: when he holds up a yellow card—to indicate that his tension is about to erupt—she holds up a corresponding yellow card, and he is off to run around the track once. Then he can settle down to his math or reading for twenty minutes."

"Isn't that a bit too permissive for a school to accept?"

"They may think so, but a child ought to have some options within the rules. The rule is *go to school,* but there should be some freedom for children to learn according to their own special way or speed."

New Wives' Tale: Beating a child for poor school performance is like scolding him for getting the mumps.

"If you want to learn anything, you must sit still, keep your mouth shut, and listen."

"My eight-year-old boy is one of those hyperactive children. He has trouble sitting still and listening. He is learning, he likes school, his reading is up to grade level, but his third-grade teacher is rather strict. She wants everyone to sit still and pay attention. He's okay for about twenty minutes, and then he gets restless and bored. He makes some funny crack to a friend and gets sent out to stand in the hall to think things over. Usually he makes faces out there and, of course, the class laughs —which is just more encouragement, I guess. The teacher takes it all personally and becomes simply furious. She believes we haven't taught him self-control. We really leaned on him, believe me, but he gets worse with more pressure."

"It's December now. Do you think he will pass this year before they suspend him?"

"She says he's smart enough and has learned enough, so he'll pass, but most likely he'll have unfinished work. She has to grade him on what he puts down on paper."

"Do you know the teacher he'll get next year?"

"She's even tougher. They claim he'd better learn self-discipline now, because after the fifth grade there are more independent projects, and if he doesn't shape up, he'll never make it through high school. They say his good brain will be wasted if he doesn't channel his energy into learning. I can hold him together until school is out, but when does he outgrow this problem?"

"If he keeps this up and they keep it up, he will begin to hate school and do some foolish antisocial act that will get him thrown out. Or he will eventually just drop out and turn off all academic pursuits. Most of the dropouts and drug freaks I see in adolescence were restless kids in grade school who got put down just because they were hyperactive or bored or had dyslexia. If they are called 'bad' long enough, they begin to believe it and act badly."

"I know all that. Give me a practical solution *now.*"

"Is there an 'open' school or private school where you could send him? Doing work on a contract basis, each child competes with himself only. Usually the classes are smaller and the distractions are fewer, although in some open classes the noise and activity levels are so high that these children get worse."

"There is one, but it's expensive and I'd have to drive him there."

"Maybe you could afford the tuition for one year just to get away from the overly restrictive atmosphere. The headmaster of a Pennsylvania school told me about his rather successful experiment. The teacher-pupil ratio is one to ten, which is a help right there. On Monday, each child fills out a contract for the week's work. The best part of this school is that each child is an expert in something, no matter how insignificant. Only one can carry messages, one runs the projector, one gets to erase all the boards, one makes gelatin, one is in charge of faculty coffee, and so on. One terribly hyperactive boy posed a problem. They finally discovered that he was an expert tree climber, so he was called from the class whenever a kite or kitten needed retrieval. The headmaster would announce over the PA system: 'There is a cat in the north oak tree. Will Tommy come and help get him down?' Tommy would run to his locker and get on his sneakers and a special T-shirt with a big 'T' on the front, the band would get their instruments, and the whole student body would assemble on the front lawn and cheer Tommy on. He really climbed well, and when he brought the errant cat down, the band would be playing some rousing Sousa march. Much acclaim followed. 'Right on!' 'You're great, Tommy.' 'Good work, Tom.' The teacher would pat him on the back: 'Very good, Tommy. Now how about a little math?' And because he felt so good about himself, he'd settle down for a day or two. When he began to disrupt the class again, the teacher would call the headmaster on the room phone: 'Tommy's at it again.' The headmaster would take his cat out of his office, shoo it up in the tree again, and get on the PA system."

"He developed the idea that every child in the school should be a winner; everyone was needed and wanted. The whole school was turned on. The principal usually sets the tone of the school. Talk to this present one to see if he is interested in trying something innovative. We've got to hold your son together until he outgrows this."

"I can't change the school system!"

"I'll help. We'll work out a plan. You know, there are other ways children can learn. Just because 80 percent do well in the traditional fashion is no reason the other 20 percent must shape up and fit into that mold. Many new electronic devices have been helpful in education. In our state, children with dyslexia can use records and tapes made for the blind. A child can learn through his ears while he is getting remedial reading. If he has to make out a report, he can dictate it into a tape recorder and a mother can type it for him. It's still *his* work, although the pathway was ear-brain-mouth. Why does it *have* to be eyes-brain-fingers? How about supplying a disruptive, hyperactive child with a cassette and earpiece, and let him learn his lessons while running around the school athletic field or riding a bike or horse? He could come in when the lesson was over, take a test, get a new cassette and be off. He wouldn't bug the teacher nor disrupt the class, and he might be learning something."

New Wives' Tale: If Edison had not been thrown out of school, we might be still using candles.

"If you want your child to have the right friends, you should choose them yourself."

"I don't want to be too meddlesome, but I don't like the friend my ten-year-old son brings home from school. Is there anything I can do without getting everyone mad at me?"

"Geography has a lot to do with friends. You could move, but things might be worse. What's your boy's friend like?"

"He's loud, boisterous, bossy. He wants to organize everything. My boy seems to enjoy being directed or manipulated."

"Maybe at this time of his life he needs that. Remember Romeo and Juliet? The more the parents tried to separate them, the closer they got. To a certain extent you cannot fight their friendship. Maybe you could join it."

"What do you mean?"

"Great decisions are made by people who figured out a problem by themselves, or thought they did. Your son might be embarrassed by this boy's behavior if you invited him for dinner with the family or if you all went to the movies together."

"What if they get along beautifully?"

"Then you may have to be tolerant of a life style that you are not comfortable with."

"There must be a better, quicker way."

"Proscribing contact sometimes works. But you cannot protect your child from the world. How much better to allow him to make an error—if it is one—in the safety of your acceptance than to find out about the awful world at age eighteen. Lecturing almost never works; he must really experience human contacts by experiencing human contacts."

"He's just like my husband: picking up every stray dog in the street."

"Maybe it's genetic."

New Wives' Tale: A burned child dreads fire. Roll, don't push.

"If he doesn't go to college, he'll be a failure."

"My son is a junior in high school and his grade point has slipped down to 2.5. If he doesn't straighten out he'll never make it to college. He's not a great athlete so he won't get in on some scholarship. He used to be so smart. Has he got mono? Could you find out if he's taking drugs?"

"Maybe he doesn't want to go to college. Are you and your husband eager for him to go?"

"Oh, yes. We both went and think he should also. I'm afraid my husband will be keenly disappointed if he doesn't make it. Isn't there a pill that would turn him on?"

"Do you think he is being noncompliant because you're pushing college? Some adolescents do just the opposite of what we think is best for them. Maybe he thinks he can't live up to the standards of his parents."

"Oh, he's as smart as we are. We've always told him, 'You're a smart boy; you'll do well in college.' "

"Maybe he's not so sure. Maybe he needs some time to figure out who he is and what he wants."

"We've told him if he gets good grades and stays out of trouble he can go into any profession he wants."

"That may be just what he is dragging his feet about. He's seen Boeing and Lockheed engineers out of jobs. He's heard that there are ten college graduates for every one position in medical and law schools—and they all have close to 4.0 grade point averages. He may not only think he can't make it but if he does, he won't be any better for it. What *does* he like to do?"

"Cars, motors, and drums."

"Sounds like fun. You may have to accept those interests as his. Why don't you try the gimmick of encouraging those activities, and then if he grows bored he'll move on to something he is more comfortable in?"

"Nothing more we can do?"

"Not now, but save your money. If he has good native intelligence he may yet get to college. At least for now let him make up his own mind. Ask him what he wants to do. Suggest a year or two of work after high school. Get off his back."

New Wives' Tale: If your child grows up to be happier than you, he may also be smarter.

8

"The Pediatrician Treats Only Children"

You're a new pediatrician, and your very first patient is a five-week-old baby who seems normal and healthy. His mother wants a few answers.

"I change his diapers twenty times a day. Is that too much?"

"Does he have twenty B.M.'s a day?"

"No, I just like to keep him fresh and clean."

You try to remember if anything was ever said in medical school about diapers, but you draw a blank. So you sit, nod your head, and give the standard, "hmmm."

"Why don't you cut down to eighteen or nineteen for a while?"

You wonder why they don't get typhoid; you'd really be ready for *that.*

The next patient is another healthy month-old in for the first checkup. "You're doing fine. Any questions?"

The mother is not sure of one thing. "I don't particularly enjoy diaper changing. Is it okay to change him only three times a day?"

You are now a diaper expert. The oracle speaks: "Some people change diapers three times a day; some find it best for them to change diapers twenty times a day. The majority of parents change the diapers between three and twenty times—when wet and/or dirty. If you and the baby are comfortable, then you are probably changing at the proper frequency."

The parents are impressed with your knowledge. They take notes as you speak. Because they nod their heads as you talk, you feel that you have hit on a universal truism and file it away with other cheerful facts to be retrieved with the next diaper question.

Doctors are virtually forced to abide by one of Parkinson's laws: If you are asked a question, you must answer it. Because the patient has chosen you as her doctor, you are loath to antagonize her, so your advice usually is a compromise between what the patient is doing and what you—the doctor—consider proper.

If you had smirked, snickered, or even raised an eyebrow at the twenty-diaper-a-day parent, you might have raised doubts about her adequacy or fostered guilt or even anger. The parents might have gone elsewhere at a time when you needed the business. For this reason, pediatricians (psychiatrists and internists, too) tend to become somewhat permissive in accepting different life styles. Sometimes we are called communists or even wishy-washy.

We were trained as health care specialists. Do we have a right to answer questions not related strictly to sickness? Are we obliged to invade the home to assure an optimal environment? We have laws to isolate the open tuberculosis patient from his family. Can we extend this to remove a depressed, or violent, or unloving parent from his children? Are we our patients' keepers?

A grandmother writes me from Kansas, "My son is a sergeant stationed in California. He is married to an Oriental girl and I don't think she is caring for my grandchildren properly. When I last visited them, one boy had a draining ear, one boy seemed awfully pale and listless, and she is letting the thirteen-year-old girl take tub baths during her menstrual periods. I've heard that is a good way to get tuberculosis. Please write him and give them some health tips. Sincerely, Mrs. ———. P.S. Don't tell him I told you to write; he may think I'm interfering."

How does one solve this? How about, "Dear Sergeant: It has come to my attention that . . ."? Impossible. We love to help people, but we are not supposed to make them paranoid. I wrote the Kansas grandmother suggesting she urge her son to see his local medical officer.

An aunt of a patient calls to say her sister is bringing in her niece for a checkup, but she would like me to know that her sister screams and hollers at her girl, hits her if she doesn't obey, or eat, or go to bed, or to the toilet on command. "I'm sure you can straighten things out. Oh, don't tell her I called."

So when she comes in I play it cool. The girl is the usual noncompliant two-year-old. I do most of the exam on my knees with the girl on her mother's lap. She kicks and yells "No!" The exam is okay.

I try an open-end question. "How are you two getting along? She is the usual snarly two-year-old here; what does she act like at home?"

"Okay, I guess," the mother answers wearily. "She is pretty stubborn and I raise my voice, but I suppose that's normal."

I finally dig in. "Is it fun to take care of her? Are you

depressed? Doesn't anyone hold you together?" Tears and a flood of marital and in-law problems come pouring out. I'm used to children's tears but get uncomfortable when *adults* cry; I feel silly saying, "There, there."

I get the feeling that this mother is depressed and looks on this child as the hurdle to her own happiness. Somehow I have to hold her together so she can hold her child together.

Phone call: "My once normal three-year-old now awakens screaming at about midnight. We soothe and rock him back to sleep. He happily goes off to nursery school the next day. Is it a nightmare? Is school too much? He has had all his teeth for a while."

Restlessness at night in a child who has friends is usually due to a pinworm infestation, a social disease among children. Kids with worms are often sullen, snarly, and/or tired; they may not get the best out of school. Nursery school, kindergarten, and early grade school teachers should organize pinworm group therapy sessions every few months. Perhaps a room mother could plan a party with some punch suitably laced with the therapeutic syrup.

In our area the water comes from melted snow. The people suffer from a high rate of decayed, missing, and filled teeth because of the lack of fluoride. Despite many educational campaigns, the people and the legislature refuse to allow this essential ingredient into the water supply. During an unsuccessful effort to do something about the rotten teeth, I received a "personal" postcard: "Dear Doctor Smith: Didn't you know that the Russians put fluoride in the water of their satellite countries to keep them in dull submission? My brother in the C.I.A. told me this. If you are *still* for fluoride in the water you are a RED. Sincerely, ———."

We suffer these hostilities by silently clenching our teeth, which are more gold than enamel by now. If the communists nibble us to death, it will be our fault.

"My son cut his finger badly on a sharp piece of metal on a toy we got him for Christmas. We had to see a surgeon; he said it was close to a tendon. What can we do? The toy was labeled as being appropriate for his age."

"Be sure to write the manufacturer; they need to know. Also call the state consumer protection agency and complain. We have to do something about dangerous toys."

"My child fell off the jungle gym at the school playground and was knocked out. He's okay now, but they just recently covered the grass with blacktop. Didn't they think kids would fall down on this?"

"School administrators feel that it is safer than coming into the slippery halls with mud and/or grass on the shoes and falling on the harder floors. Maybe you could form a protection and safety committee in the P.T.A. and provide a safer, somewhat flexible play surface, and/or carpeting in the halls." One would think the schools could design nonlethal play areas.

Must we do everything? The American Academy of Pediatrics is heavily committed as the child's advocate. Various pressure groups and committees are trying to influence legislation to standardize seat restraints that work, to forbid the use of lead paint on interior surfaces, to cut down salt and sugar in infants' food. Reducing so much violence in TV and comics has been a recent concern. Dr. Spock may be on to something; by showing children violence, we may be suggesting it as a way of life.

"Doctor, do you take welfare children as patients?

We now have a six-year-old foster child and I would like you to take care of him just as you do our own. He cannot understand why he must be taken to the medical school clinic when the rest of us have our own doctor. He's been put down so much I'm afraid he will be more convinced than ever that he is no good."

Most of us take our share of children on welfare even though we cannot pay the office expenses with what the welfare services allow. Our government's priorities seem all screwed up.

"I'd like to have rooming-in but the hospital says it's against the rules. My obstetrician seems afraid to deliver me at home; in case something goes wrong, he'd like to have the emergency facilities."

"He's got a point; don't put him in an uncomfortable position or you may not get his optimum care. Let me tell you what a patient of mine did and see if you like it. It was this family's third baby. She went to the hospital when the labor pains began, delivered fairly routinely, was put to bed, and slept soundly all night. When her doctor was making rounds the next day and found her recovering satisfactorily, she told him she would like to be discharged. He was reluctant, as he preferred a three-day postpartum stay. She was adamant and said she would call a doctor if something happened. She signed out and left with her husband, who checked in with her and the rest of the family at a nearby motel. They had a catered steak dinner that night, she breastfed her baby on demand, she could play with her other children. It was a pleasant vacation, but it's not for everyone."

One would think the hospitals would get the message that they are supposed to serve the people. They sometimes act as if the patients are upsetting their routine.

Studies have shown that there is a better mother-child reaction and mutuality if the mother and child can be closer from birth on. The premie is a special problem, but some interaction can be worked out even with the baby in the incubator; the mother should be allowed to reach through and touch *her* child. Something is forever lost if she is sent home and then called in a month with, "Your baby is ready."

"What baby? Oh, yes, now I remember."

Father calls. "He's been a juvenile delinquent ever since he tried to flush his bottle down the toilet at age one. Well, he's really blown it this time. My jerky son, age fourteen, didn't have a history assignment in on time. The teacher called him on it and he called her a dirty word. I guess she had had enough of him so she sent him to the principal, who suspended him. He can come back if he apologizes and we take him somewhere for counseling. He won't do the former and I can't afford the latter. Do we kill him now or let the cops do it later when he robs a bank, because that's where he's heading."

Everyone has had a crack at the boy. The psychiatrist made the parents feel guilty. The psychologist found a normal IQ but an ego crippled with hostility toward authority. His pediatrician tried amphetamines, with temporary benefit. His teachers said he could do the work if he would try; he was in the ninth grade, but with a reading level of grade three or four. He was able to fake it for a while, but after the sixth grade, with so much of education depending on reading he fell irrevocably behind. He was alternately embarrassed, miserable, angry, bitter, depressed. His parents stood over him and shouted, and the teachers cited him as an example to the class. The worst blow of all came from his peer group who called him "stupid," "jerk," "slob."

He hated himself and found solace with other losers, skipping school, swiping records and food, and "borrowing" cars. When caught, they seemed to enjoy the attention and acted as if they had no conscience. They frequently vandalized their school, a natural reaction as it was the cause of their frustration. Ask any principal. He has the names of the five to ten nonacademic boys whom he calls in when windows are broken.

It is all so unnecessary. Such a waste. Well-documented statistics indicate that 50 percent of boys who are truant from school and steal become felons in later life. Why do they skip school? Because they are unsuccessful—it's that easy. We have to allow them to be successful. School has to be fun.

We have new methods of teaching the nonreader to read, and there are now medicines to hold the hyperactive in his seat. Making parents guilty, making fun of the already embarrassed child, are counterproductive. Grounding him for underachieving will only motivate him to escape.

"My son, age fifteen, is a little heavy and nonathletic but P.E. is required and I was hoping he would get some good out of it. Today in the mail I got a notice that he is skipping gym. I knew he didn't like it, but I didn't think he would fail to show up. He's usually very conscientious. What's the matter?"

This is not unusual. In the locker room the boy sees that 90 percent of the other boys have adult-sized genitalia. He knows they are making fun of his abdominal fat, his ten puny pubic hairs, and a penis a toy poodle would be ashamed of. Of course he's going to avoid the whole P.E. program because he has to undress and take a shower. If I don't write an excuse for him, he will quit school. Whoever made up the school P.E. rules must be a mesomorphic jock who matured in one week at age thirteen between grade school and high school. Most of the rest of us had to struggle with our odd hormonal changes for years and were terribly embarrassed.

"I don't understand my daughter. Would you recommend a psychologist or psychiatrist for us to go to?"

You're an experienced pediatrician so you dig around: "What's the matter?"

"She's fifteen years old and either crying about some minor problem or angry because I said some innocuous thing to her."

"Maybe I ought to check her out first." She had just recovered from mononucleosis; she was mildly anemic; she was having stomach aches and headaches from a milk, chocolate, wheat, and eggs diet; and her self-image was down because she had gained seven pounds. A little manipulation of the diet, a few medicines, some encouragement and time, and she was okay. A psychiatrist or psychologist would have assumed that all the metabolic, infectious, parasitic, and endocrine problems had been solved and her problem was a family imbalance or at least an environmental stress. Of course, they would have found such a psychological problem; there are always a few around.

New Wives' Tale: A pediatrician is a scientific grandmother who should be allowed to straighten out the world.

9

Mothers and Fathers

Old Wives' Tale: "Have a baby; save the marriage."

"I don't know if you can help me but I have to start somewhere. You've been helping me rear my two-year-old and he's been a delight up to now. All at once he's a whiney, surly, stubborn handful. Almost at the same time I find my husband has become a whiney, surly, stubborn 25-year-old. I'd like to get him involved with the care and discipline, but the more I try, the more excuses he finds for working late and going on business trips. My mother thinks I should have another baby and he would come back to the nest again. It would be very simple to stop the pills for a couple of days."

"Was he helpful two years ago when this one was a baby?"

"He was okay, but I had to do most everything—he seemed so clumsy."

"Maybe he feels left out. The baby may have come between you, like a lover."

"Oh, dear! I didn't mean to let that happen. I thought

I was doing him a favor by doing all the feeding and changing."

"We all need to feel needed or wanted. He may have just drifted away. That delightful age from two to eight months is the time to get a husband really involved with a baby's care. Babies that age smile and laugh and usually love to be cuddled. If a father can feed, change, bathe, and dress a baby and get smiled at, he usually gets 'trapped' into really feeling he is useful. It may not be too late. Maybe he can be persuaded to have an outing with your son when both are not crabby, tired, or hungry; he might just get hooked into wanting to be a father again."

"Well, I'll try, but I don't know."

"For God's sake, though, don't stop your pills. Having another baby might really push him out of the nest."

New Wives' Tale: A baby is a poor marriage counselor.

"Father earns a living; Mother rears the kids."

"It's really no fun for me. My five-year-old is becoming a behavior problem; I'm getting depressed with a stomach ache that alternates with a headache and insomnia. I don't think I can hold together much longer."

"What does your husband do?"

"He drives a truck and earns the money to feed and clothe us. He feels his responsibility ends there. He feels that I'm supposed to be satisfied with the home and the child he has provided. Don't get me wrong. I love my husband; he's kind and gentle and a good provider. It just seems he'd rather drive than stay home."

"Have you reminded him he has some domestic obligations?"

"Yes, but he says he must take on extra jobs so he can

provide for us and have some savings for the boy's education."

"Any other interests of his?"

"Some sports and bowling; I'm sure there's no other woman, if that's what you mean."

"Does he like the boy?"

"He used to adore him, but he simply can't find the time to spend with him any more. I have the feeling that our home isn't such a great place to be, so he finds his work much more satisfying."

"Can *you* get out of the house?"

"To the store and to see a neighbor occasionally."

"Do you have enough energy to get a part-time job while your son is in school? It just might get you out of your rut."

"I know I should, but my husband thinks it's some kind of insult to him as the head of the house if the male can't take care of the family."

"That's a lot of bull. He learned that from the last generation. Women's Lib has at least pointed out that *both* parents are caretakers and providers. You two have to have a good discussion about life goals and fulfillment, or you should see a marriage counselor."

"I touched on this once and he seemed hurt. He can't see why I'm not satisfied. But by the way, why *aren't* I satisfied?"

"You may be constitutionally depressed or at least disappointed because your early hopes haven't been realized. Can you get your husband involved with your son somehow? Fishing, bowling, something? Most sons are delighted when their fathers show them what they do all day. Could he help change a tire, load a truck, check invoices, or whatever they do? I'll bet some of the boy's undesirable behavior will improve once someone pays attention to him and lets him believe he's needed and wanted. Seeing your boy cheer up will cheer you up, and your husband might think home is fun again. And if you have a job, you might find something more interesting to talk about than the noise in the washer."

New Wives' Tale: If you don't enjoy taking care of another human being, it won't work.

Not so long ago we all were convinced that the female was the key figure in child-rearing. It was her egg that became fertilized, her uterus that nurtured the fetus, her straining that delivered it, and her breast milk that made it grow. In that first year she really seemed to be turned on to this baby. She laughed and played with it and seemed completely wrapped up in his welfare. When asked how she felt, her response was an unequivocal, "This is the best time of my life."

Even though she complained of backache and fatigue, it all seemed to be so much fun that husbands and in-laws assumed this was the reason for her whole existence, and once she launched her child into school it was time to fill her uterus again. Back in farming and fishing and hunting days it all seemed so natural that the woman should be intimately involved with the babies.

This was a neat picture of the young, struggling family—each parent using innate skills to provide for the home. The child would grow up to assume his rightful place, a boy like his father and a girl like her mother. Everyone was wanted and needed. Children were needed because there was no insurance or social security to care for the aged. There were fewer aged also; few adults lived past forty or fifty years.

As the mother was the parent in charge of upbringing, she was a convenient scapegoat if the child did not fit in or was spoiled or noncompliant or just different or strange.

Each child files away in his memory feelings, attitudes, thoughts, sounds, and sights which, right or wrong, he has learned from his parents. He internalizes his parents in such a way that they continue to influence him despite death or distance. If he sees his mother working in the house and father in the field, he imprints this as a universal truism, like gravity. When he matures, he tries to organize his life to perpetuate this concept. Anything else causes anxiety.

Our society has changed—with inventions, technology, and communication—but our concept of the family and parental roles cannot. It takes about three generations to change parental attitudes about role-playing.

Therefore, I was a little upset some years ago when my wife awakened me at 2:00 A.M. suggesting that I might feed our month-old baby, who was screaming lustily in the next room. She said she was tired, she didn't have any more breast milk, and if I was to be any help to new mothers, maybe I should get up and feed the baby myself.

I said I had learned all that in school and isn't a woman supposed to take care of children and what if the neighbors saw me? Other cogent reasons fell on deaf ears. In my usual cool, scientific approach I heated some milk to what seemed body temperature and aimed it at the open mouth in the crib. The milk rapidly disappeared. I tried to remain detached so I wouldn't wake up completely and would be able to return to sleep easily. I changed her. A tap on her upper left abdomen suggested swallowed air. I rolled her on her right side, patted her a few times, sat her up and she thanked me with a burp and a big smile. I'm a human being, and when someone smiles at me, I smile back.

She didn't know who I was, but she figured I saved her life; a complete stranger passing in the middle of the night. I wondered then how she knew what to do. Some gene for smiling must exist in the human like the blinking, crying, sucking reflexes. Eons ago it must have allowed for survival as the smiling baby was fed (was the crying, constantly fussy baby discarded?) and a mutuality developed: "I'll feed you if you smile at me."

Although I didn't know it there at 2:00 A.M., I had stumbled on a universal truth: a human enjoys helping another human if he knows what to do and is rewarded in some way for doing it. It raises his self-esteem if he feels needed; maybe the real reason for having children is to feel needed and wanted. I began to look forward to these nightly sessions and would even awaken and have the bottle ready so the poor thing would not have to wait so long. Pretty soon her smiles would interfere with her swallowing and milk would ooze out of the corner of her mouth.

My wife, not insensitive to the goings-on, would call out, "What are you two doing in there?"

"Nothing. Just a little father-daughter interaction."

However, it *was* getting to be a little bit of a drag, so I gradually reduced the quantity of milk over the next week and our daughter began to sleep through.

But we were both hooked. I had filed away in my temporal lobe memory center that if my daughter wanted anything in the middle of the night and smiled, I would be ready with the answer to her request. She learned that if she smiled she could get almost anything. Now, 23 years later, she calls every few weeks from college—usually at night—and asks for not milk, but money. She knows I cannot refuse because I have been programmed to respond. She also knows that I want to comply quickly so I can get back to sleep. I am now awaiting the arrival of some nice young man to take my place in her scheme of things; someone who will feed and comfort her and otherwise take care of her in the middle of the night.

This is a form of prejudice, of course. My mother learned that the role of a woman was to take care of her husband, the children, and the house. She must have done this because she had been taught to. She was comfortable doing it or would have felt guilty if she had not, or didn't know she had any other option. Having observed this in my mother, I was surprised to find my wife frequently beating me out of the house in the morning. Being a nurse, conducting an art tour, going to a board meeting seemed to excite her almost as much as caring for the wonderful children I had allowed her to bear for me. Even after I blessed her with five children, she seemed to be *more* determined to get out of the house. It didn't make sense; the more children, the more she wanted to go to work. But this regime seemed to be successful for her, because she is intelligent, is well organized, and has a high energy level. She made nourishing breakfasts (always served with cloth napkins), made the beds (until the children were old enough to make them themselves), started the wash, oriented the sitter, all before she left. The children got quality care. She also found she didn't have to sit all day worrying if their thumb-sucking, bed-rocking, bottom-clutching, whining behavior meant insecurity.

It took me years to figure how much healthier an influence this was on the children and the collective domestic sanity. The children look on her now as a person with rights and feelings, and not as a faucet to be turned on. She has kept abreast of the community and has vital, compelling interests that will permit her to feel needed long after our children are no longer dependent. Our children also feel less guilty as they leave home. I have the feeling that she will not miss me so much—my mother was left with little but emptiness and self-pity for twenty years after Dad died.

New Wives' Tale: If it isn't fun it won't work.

"Children should be seen and not heard."

"My husband talks to clients all day, so when he gets home he wants peace and quiet. The children are crabby, screaming and fighting. He gets mad and may even spank them. Dinner is a shambles. No one can eat and we are all crying. I'd like to dump the whole thing and go to some Pacific island. Is there a way out?"

"I'd like to say it's worms or anemia, but I can't use those excuses all the time. Somehow you have to change the routine. The children may have discovered that they get some attention from their father by being obnoxious."

"He's so mean I would think they'd learn to shut up when he gets home."

"Kids want attention; it doesn't seem to matter if it's good or bad. I'm sure the worse they get, the worse he gets. Why don't you try a change: feed them a light snack about a half hour before he gets home—in case low blood sugar is the problem. Then, while they're at the table, have them draw a picture or write a two-line poem or something. When your husband comes in, let him sit down and stare into space for a minute, and then have the children go in one at a time and present their productions to him singly. He might need a drink of sherry, but if this doesn't turn him on to the delights of fatherhood, then maybe you'd better find out who's putting him down at the office. He may be so depressed about his life that he can't give of himself to anyone else. Who holds *you* together?"

"I get a few kicks from bowling and the church, but I often have a tightness in my stomach at home."

New Wives' Tale: We* all *need to be seen and heard.

"Don't let a child see you cry."

"My father died last Monday and the funeral is tomorrow. My five-year-old son was very close to him. My mother and I cannot decide if he should be allowed to come to the funeral or not. He wants to come, but he doesn't know what it will be like."

"Does he know that his grandfather is gone?"

"We've told him that Grandpa has gone to heaven and that he will never see him again. But he knows Grandfather will be there and he insists on going. Mother says, 'No,' but I'm not sure."

"I'm not sure either. If he was very close to his grandfather, he may be unable to accept his death unless he is allowed to see the body and then to mourn."

"He'll cry if he goes. I'm sure I'm going to and I won't be of much help to him."

"Maybe he should cry. Maybe he should realize grandfather is really gone. Maybe he won't believe it unless he sees it."

"Maybe if we don't talk about it, it all might go away."

"It doesn't work out that way. We all have to work out our losses. He has to know, also, that you have accepted your loss, or he won't be able to accept it. It's going to drain you all but it will be better in the end."

New Wives' Tale: Children should learn when it is appropriate to laugh and when it is appropriate to cry.

"Spare the rod and spoil the child."

Research has proven that almost everything a child experiences in his life is filed away in the temporal lobe of the brain. "Gravity works," "fires burn," "knives cut," "freeways kill," "water moistens" are learned phenomena which we store as universal truth. Deep hypnosis or electrostimulation of the temporal lobe can elicit these forgotten experiences. A probe in one area of this cortex will make an adult recall, as an example, a circus he visited at age four. He can see the animals, smell the popcorn, hear the band, and even relive the excitement of the trapeze act. In a similar way, attitudes about the self are incorporated into a child's scheme of things; it is society's way of internalizing a method of impulse control so the adult can function as a social animal.

The mother deer nurses her fawn, who learns to trust its mother (who else?). He is prejudiced to believe her rules of behavior, which are primarily for survival. She disciplines the fawn for danger. "Look out for the puma!" This is a universal deer truth. She probably doesn't have time to worry or nag about sloppy eating habits, defecating in the water hole, or other insignificant actions nonessential to survival.

The human animal is also exploring his dangerous

world and finds some painful limits; hot fire, sharp objects, scary baths, constant pull of gravity, and so on. In addition, however, a number of his actions, he finds, are punishable by his loving parents. Emotional pain or fear of loss of parental love is as compelling to his awareness of the world as is broken glass.

Disapproval for not going right to sleep, for not having a bowel movement on the toilet on command, for sucking his thumb after age ten months, for rocking the bed, for wetting the bed after age four or five, for messing in his food, for whining—all are stored by the child as memories and attitudes about himself adjacent to information about danger in the world. He therefore will believe that he is not especially worthwhile because many normal infantile growth or developmental traits were looked on as "bad" and thus remembered. (Ignoring them would serve to extinguish most of them before they became emotionally fortified and a part of an overwhelming conscience in adulthood.) He learns he is not acceptable to his parents and thus acquires this same attitude about himself, which he carries with him long after his parents are no longer part of his physical environment.

From my Baltimore-reared mother I learned that blacks were okay but somehow should be considered servile. I have been a little shaken to meet many blacks who were not willing to accept this label and who expected to be treated as equals and not as stereotypes. It has taken me years to unlearn "Eenie-meeny-minie-mo; catch a nigger by the toe."

Foreigners observing the American scene criticize our prejudices, but witness the depth of suspicion and hatred the Irish have for the British. Many Scots would just as soon build up Hadrian's wall again. Swedes think the Finns are Mongol peasants. Russian children have been taught to hate the Germans; but what would you have said to your children in 1945 if another country had killed 25 million of your own people? What are Israeli parents saying to their children about the Egyptians, and vice versa? It is not the leaders of these countries who lead their people to war, but the citizens' temporal lobes which virtually force them into battle.

Sociologists estimate it takes about three generations to wipe out prejudice. Governments, churches, and the various media can provide the laws, the words, and the institutions to defuse the destructive attitudes. A family might not be so lucky in preventing the perpetuation of a poor self-image. A parent who beats a child for sucking his thumb or for "just standing there" frequently rears a child who hates himself and looks on his own children as targets for his own dissatisfaction. As in a fraternity initiation, if it is okay for the sophomore to haze the freshman, it is acceptable for the same beaten ones to become the beaters the next year.

A healthy interruption to this self-perpetuating hostility has been initiated by Mayor Charles Evers of Fayette, Mississippi, who fines any black for calling a white a "honky" or any white for calling a black a "nigger." "You have to start someplace," he says. He has an ordinance against selling and eating watermelon on the street—a personal prejudice relating to the days when he and his brother Medgar were *made* to eat watermelon and dance in the street by white folk who threw pennies at them—a race putdown which helped to perpetuate the myth of white supremacy.

It may take three generations of busing to show the

whites that the black pigment does not rub off. The churches are trying to do more than sermonize "Love thy neighbor" and "Be nice to one another." You cannot be nice to another human being unless you like yourself first. Psychosurgery destroys too much of the brain to be effective yet. Psychoanalysis is too costly and time-consuming to get around to all of us.

Somehow we have to program our children to feel that we *want* them; it's too bad that we cannot indicate that we *need* them also. We have to stop punishing behavior that is a part of growing up. Psychologists and pediatricians have got to get the message out that we must first establish mutual trust and then discipline for danger. It is *not* dangerous to be diapered until you are two or three years old. It is *not* dangerous to suck your thumb until your kindergarten peers laugh you out of it. It may be dangerous for a parent and a child to be separated by the mechanics of running an obstetrical service. It is dangerous for a father to think he is not a parent and therefore cannot participate in the child's care.

New Wives' Tale: Do spoil, but call it "programming for mutual trust."

"Children of divorced parents are insecure."

"My husband and I are getting a divorce and I know my five-year-old boy is going to fall apart. I've tried to hold the marriage together for his sake, but things are impossible."

"Some children do better with one parent or in a home with less fighting. How do you know he will disintegrate?"

"He's such a nervous, restless, sensitive child already. He can't relax and sleep at night, he can't eat a decent meal, he talks all the time, he laughs easily and cries easily—shall I go on?"

"No, you've told me enough so that I get the message he is somewhat hyperactive."

"Oh, that brain problem that bothers them in school? I thought all those things meant he came from an unhappy home."

"Lots of kids come from homes where there is strife; many of them really don't care as long as they know someone will be taking care of them. Hyperactive children notice their environment more and respond to it physically. Did you really think you made him this way?"

"Who else? I feel so guilty that I didn't love him enough—but he was difficult to cuddle and threw up a lot."

"Well, I should have emphasized that years ago. That's the way he's built, and the genes that make him that way usually come from the father. What is his father like?"

"That's why we're getting a divorce. He won't nest. It's, 'Let's do this; let's do that,' until I could scream. He has two jobs; he seems to like work more than his home. We have a nice house, I've kept my figure, and we have no sex hangups. But I'm not going to rear this child all alone; I married a man, not an idea."

"Tell me about your husband's early school years."

"He hated school. Repeated a grade. He's very bright but couldn't or didn't do his work. Wait a minute! I see what you're leading up to. I'd always thought that my son learned to be restless because he observed his father; but he was never around enough to observe. You are telling me that he inherited this trait."

"Heredity must account for at least 50 to 70 percent

of hyperactive boys. The ratio of hyperactive boys to girls is about seven or eight to one which suggests hereditary factors."

New Wives' Tale: A man with a short attention span may not be able to remain married very long.

10

"As the Twig Is Bent . . ."

Old Wives' Tale: "A child who sucks his thumb is insecure and will grow up to be a neurotic or a criminal."

"My child was three years old yesterday and his thumb-sucking has got to stop. I know he's insecure because he whines all the time, but his dentist says he'll need braces until he's married, and my mother-in-law says I'm a failure as a mother or I would have made him stop long ago. I'm frantic. I shout at him and slap his hand, but that only works for about ten minutes. What can I do? I've heard if I put asafetida on his thumb he might quit."

"Psychiatrists might say that he is fixed at the oral level because he didn't get enough satisfaction at breast or bottle. Behavior therapists might say that he has learned to suck because he is rewarded with attention for doing it. Somehow I have to get you to stop worrying about it. If I reassured you about the habit, would you or could you stop pestering him about it?"

"I'm not sure. Before I had children I promised myself I'd never have a child who had a snotty nose or sucked his thumb. That's exactly what I've got."

"Did you or your husband suck as children?"

"We both did. I did until age six; my husband until ten."

"I'm sure there must be a gene for thumb-sucking, and it runs strongly in your family. Also, your mother probably bugged you about it, so you have strong built-in feelings regarding it."

In 1911 a child care expert announced to the world that any child who sucked his thumb would grow up to be a criminal. At that time the new theories of adult neurosis suggested that infantile drives, if frustrated, would lead directly to adult psychopathology. If a child were subjected to poor parenting, he might remain fixed at some emotional level—oral, anal, or genital. He could grow physically and intellectually, but not emotionally.

A thumb-sucking child was a case in point: obviously he was insecure or he would not have to cling to this oral gratification for such a long time. An insecure person would be unable to cope with the realities of life so would retreat to infantile methods of handling anxiety.

An alcoholic was assumed to be "fixed" at the oral level: the drink made him feel warm and good; he married a woman older than he; when inebriated his dependency upon her to tuck him in bed, clean up his messes, and forgive him was a reliving of the oral stage from which he was unable to progress.

The fat cook chose his life's work because of his oral drives.

If a child at age two were psychologically hurt, he might become anal-retentive. As an adult he would be obsessive-compulsive, withholding, a nit-picking string-saver.

Don Juan might be said to have been thwarted in working out his Oedipal hangups at age five or six. Homosexuality is supposed to have had its roots in a disturbed sexual identification at this early age.

All abnormal behavior was assumed to be a distortion of an individual's ability to handle anxiety. Find the block, remove it, and the patient should find a healthy, socially acceptable method of handling anxiety.

It became patently obvious that this assumed connection between an infantile habit and adult psychopathology was false. Some statistic gathering following this 1911 prediction indicated that although something like 40 percent of infants and children sucked their thumbs, criminals did not constitute 40 percent of the population. Just about as many thumb-suckers grew up to be "straight" as grew up to be criminals.

Some damage was done, however, because parents who believed this was so began an all out frontal attack on the symptom. When they became convinced that thumb-sucking was a "bad" thing, they fought it. Elbow cuffs were devised to prevent easy access of thumb to mouth. Asafetida was painted on the thumb as aversive therapy. Children were put to bed with boxing gloves on or their hands were tied to the crib side. They were told they were "bad" and "Stop that or I'll spank you." Everything but the cattle prod was used, but the children kept on. Some transferred their oral efforts to their toes or the bed or the plaster. Some found they could suck their tongues and discovered they could make themselves vomit—which would get even more response from their angry parents.

It was as easy to stop this habit as it was to change

the color of the child's eyes. The resolute parents refused to relent, as if committed to extinguish this reminder of some "sin" imposed on the family. Moreover, many children who were called "bad" for so long began to believe they were bad and *became* bad, thus fulfilling the prophecy. Some thumb-suckers, then, did grow up to be bad or neurotic or criminals because they were told they would.

A retraction was in order to get parents to back off, but few heard it, or if they did it was too late to prevent this prejudice against thumb-sucking from becoming an established truism in child-rearing. Young parents now generally don't mind if their child sucks his thumb, but grandparents reared under the influence of the old prejudices are loath to smile and look the other way.

Grandmother calls. "I know my grandson is insecure at his own home; he didn't suck his thumb *once* while he stayed with me this last weekend. Just as soon as I took him home and he saw his mother, he stuck his thumb in his mouth. She frowned at him so he knows how she feels about him. I'd be willing to pay for a marriage counselor, or do they need a psychiatrist?"

"Everyone probably needs a psychiatrist at one time or another, but I think your daughter and son-in-law are basically doing a good job. Maybe you and I could give a little love and support. Let them know they're doing a good job and let the boy know he is loved and wanted. Everyone has feelings of insecurity. By the way, what do you do with the boy when you have him for a weekend?"

Grandmother answers: "Well, we do indulge him a little bit; we see him so seldom. We feed him, play games, read stories, go to the zoo—we never rest. He does say 'gimme,' 'mine,' and 'I want' an awful lot."

He has a different set of actions that get responses at Grandma's, so he doesn't need to suck his thumb there. He probably can't get his thumb into his candy- and gum-laden mouth anyway.

Most children are anxious to be accepted by their peer group after age four or five, so many home behaviors must be discontinued and more appropriate school behaviors substituted. Thumb-suckers may have to keep their hands in their pockets or chew on a pencil so they won't be called unflattering names by their friends, who are usually suffering from the same problems of self-control. The child runs home after school, shuts the door, and just gets his thumb in his mouth as his mother greets him, "Well, how was . . . oh, have you been sucking your thumb all day?"

"I'm home, I'm home," he thinks. He can tell by the old familiar frown on her face.

Probably the most destructive part of this overconcern is the flavor it imparts to the rest of the parent-child relationship. Parents want their children to be brave, smart, and secure, and any behavior that suggests immaturity allows them to demonstrate disappointment in their children. The parent may be upset with the behavior, but the child gets the message that he, as a person, is less than acceptable. He develops a prejudice against himself, that he is not up to some standard. He becomes depressed and discouraged and figures, "What is the point of trying?" He acquires a bad self-image.

Thumb-sucking concern, like a government bureau, is difficult to eliminate. Parental reaction to a thumb-sucking child may be more akin to racial prejudice; we may need a government edict to get parents to stop their concern. But it will take about three generations of parents to defuse this issue and a few other false, but cherished beliefs.

In an effort to give weight to the unimportance of this childhood habit, a psychologist did a retrospective study of a hundred normal adults. The fact that these adults were Air Force officers may vitiate the results of the study for some readers, but one has to assume that an Air Force officer must be reasonably free of anxiety, is fairly intelligent, and would have some trouble sucking his thumb through the oxygen mask! He also might short circuit his flight suit if he wet himself. The psychologist was able to get the childhood stories on these men and was not too surprised to learn that they all had some childhood trait that could be called a behavior problem: 40 percent sucked their thumbs, 15 percent wet the bed, 10 percent had tics or twitches, 5 percent had some school phobia, and there was a sprinkling of tantrums, impulsiveness, hair pulling, aggressiveness, headaches, stomach aches, fecal soiling, and nervousness. All had at least one symptom, but they lost their symptoms as they grew—and this with little or no therapy. The study did not mention any special child-rearing methods, but we will have to assume that in spite of a few problems these men developed a reasonably good self-image.

Another study followed children who had been brought to a child guidance clinic for a variety of behavior problems. Here again, children who had the abovementioned symptoms, in general, grew up to be reasonably law-abiding and non-neurotic. You might have guessed that *their* children had the same traits.

Thumb-sucking has no predictable significance relative to adult pathology. As soon as we parents treat it as a normal part of childhood like eating, sweating, growing, defecating, and so on, the less it will be invested with emotion.

Apparently a child has difficulty with getting up, dressing, eating, going to school, coming home, doing a few chores, playing, eating supper, watching a little TV, brushing his teeth, and going to bed. It looks easy to us, but the child looks on it as a big deal and often has to reduce anxiety by sucking his thumb, rocking the bed, or getting a stomach ache.

Some say today's children have it easier because they have heated homes, electric blankets, nourishing meals. But if they don't feel needed to draw the water, feed the animals, or help in the kitchen, they will have trouble developing some self-esteem. A parent who views his child as an economic liability will have no trouble finding some infantile behavior to carp about. Maybe the answer to the thumb-sucking problem is to have no children unless they are really needed *and* wanted. A child in a home where he finds he is a worthwhile member will have to get his hand out of his mouth if he wants to be helpful. There seems to be no deep psychological significance to thumb-sucking unless we make it so.

New Wives' Tale: A child who sucks his thumb likes to suck his thumb.

"When your child is ten months old, it's time to potty train him."

My father was a pediatrician in the good old days of 1920 to 1940. He almost threatened the eager-to-do-the-right-thing parents with, "If you don't start toilet training soon, he may never get the idea." Visions of the child wearing bulky diapers in grade school was enough to encourage the parents to prop the somewhat surprised infant on the pot immediately after each meal. This was to take advantage of the well-known gastro-colic reflex (when the stomach fills, the colon contracts and may empty). Sometimes, if he happened to be a rapid responder, the child was fed on his throne.

Many compliant, predictable children performed well and consistently, delighting their parents, who figured they would get an "A" from my Dad on their next visit. These successes were enough to encourage him to push more parents into "developing the habit."

However, a great many otherwise normal children could not get the idea and were labeled "stubborn" by their mothers, who felt some gene from the father was responsible. It is possible that another, more powerful reflex was inhibiting subject cooperation. A cold rim of steel against the buttocks can be expected to close the sphincter muscle reflexly. These uncooperative children were often left on the pot in the hopes that something would happen. Usually a pelvic paralysis short of gluteal gangrene was enough to make the child painfully uncomfortable at worst and terribly bored at best. He soon learned to hate the whole process.

Many of the originally cooperative ones, moreover, soon discovered that they had been tricked into compliance. Perhaps for one day they had been unable to dump a firm stool; the anxious concern on the mother's face suggested that they were laying golden eggs. The standard age-appropriate defiance of authority helped to solidify their resolve. Withholding was rewarded with attention. Retention helped to solidify the stool. When it *did* pass, the painful fissure suggested continued withholding; pain is a good teacher. Just as the parents had proudly announced to the doctor, the relatives, and the envious neighbors that their child was toilet trained, he became untrained and they were loath to announce a retraction. Competitive friends, feeling they were behind in the race, put more pressure on their own children to accomplish this important step toward maturity.

The trouble with this pressuring is that it sets the tone of the whole child-rearing process. Instead of a happy growth and daily discovery of new wonders, domestic life becomes a battle scene with each side trying to outmaneuver the other.

What early child experts failed to reckon with was the orderly, but individual, development of the nervous system's capabilities. The infant holds his head up before he sits; he sits before he stands; he stands before he walks. The nerves that direct the action of the muscles of urination and defecation develop last in the orderly sequence from top to bottom. Voluntary control of urine and stool elimination is possible *after* the child walks well. "Control" before this time is largely the result of the parent shoving the pot under the child when the child indicates by the characteristic red face, breath holding, and far-away look that the gastro-colic reflex is under way. There is nothing wrong with the method as long as the parents realize they have trained *themselves* to respond to certain clues. It also saves a few diapers.

My wife had a good washer and dryer, so she didn't mind the diaper bit. She also did not feel it necessary to compete with anyone on the street to toilet train early. And, she assumed that because we had a toilet in the house, the children would eventually use it. Somehow she must have indicated to our firstborn that urinating and defecating in the toilet was a fun, grown-up thing to do. At about age two this girl said to her mother, "I go pee-pee in the pot."

Mother, playfully: "You can't; it's mine."

"Me, me; I want, I want."

Mother, now really in the spirit: "It's really just for grown-ups . . ."

"I go pee-pee!"

Mother, giving in "reluctantly": "Okay, but if you wreck my toilet, it's back in the diapers."

"I be good."

This Tom Sawyer I'll-let-you-whitewash-the-fence-if-you-give-me-something approach worked for a few days until this willful child realized she was doing something *we* wanted. She gave us the ultimate in putdowns by smearing stool on the wall—her first dirty graffiti. But eventually it worked, because she was motivated and her nervous system was mature enough to cooperate with the message sent down from her brain.

New Wives' Tales: If you enjoy going to the toilet, so will your child.

The motivated child who loves and trusts his parents can be programmed to do almost anything ***if it looks like fun.***

"Words will never hurt him."

"I'm having some trouble with discipline. My two-year-old whines, hits his little sister, won't use the pot, and won't eat. I spank him, scold, and tell him he's bad, but that doesn't seem to work. Last night I tried an experiment and told him I would kill him if he didn't go to bed. He didn't and, of course, I didn't kill him. He needs discipline. What am I doing wrong?"

"You sound like the normal parent of a normal two-year-old. I believe kids practice at age two for what they'll do in adolescence. The more noncompliant he is now, the more surly and hostile at age fourteen. You may have to reduce a few pressures. Your scolding him for not using the toilet is like our bombing a country so they will accept a peace treaty; it just increases their intransigence. A psychologist told me something he tries to get parents to do, in addition to ignoring bad behavior. We all, and children especially, like attention, and children are great imitators. You are supposed to observe. 'I see you sitting down. I see you eating. You are walking from the dining room into the kitchen. You are playing with a toy.' "

"Sounds corny. What does it do?"

"He gets attention without your moralizing or making judgments. You don't put him down. In a few days or weeks he responds to this attention and because he is a natural imitator, he will begin to notice *you*. Then he will imitate you, and, if you are reasonably normal, his behavior will become reasonably normal."

"I don't throw my food on the floor. Where did he get *that?*"

"He tried it once and you paid attention. He learned to get a response."

"I haven't the strength."

"What you are doing is more exhausting. You may have to bite your tongue to make yourself remember, but it can be fun."

"I'm laughing already."

"Things you say to him are being filed away in his memory as truisms. You give him a big glass of juice; he spills it and you can get mad and say 'bad boy.' Whose fault is that? That's sabotage. He'll hate himself because he can never attain your standard. Try to praise him twice as often as you find fault with him."

New Wives' Tale: If children are told they are no good, they will grow up to believe it.

"If your child doesn't hear you, speak up."

"Would you check John's hearing? He pays no attention to me. He never comes to dinner unless I go grab him by the ears and drag him in. I tell him to brush his teeth and he doesn't."

"We can check his hearing but it sounds like domestic deafness to me."

"What's that?"

"If children hear only questions and commands, they usually turn off their parents' wavelength. Before you come in, try a little game one parent told me about. They made the diagnosis and then initiated treatment, and it was fun. The whole feeling in the home changed from degrading nit-picking to a cheerful sharing."

"Tell me; tell me."

"When they were eating at the table or reading in the living room, mother would whisper to father, 'If Carol will look in the mailbox she'll find something nice.' Carol began to listen more intently because there was always some minor goody where they said it would be. The parents were able to talk in low voices, and Carol listened to everything they said because she didn't know when it might be the clue for some treasure. They lived happily ever after. Well, for a couple of months."

New Wives' Tale: If you want your child to hear you, say something that's important to him.

"If a child has an allowance, he will learn the value of money."

"Please help settle a family argument. I want my children to understand about money by giving them an allowance. My husband says it will never work. We agreed to go by your advice."

"You put me on the spot. You may both be right. Maybe you could give one an allowance, and use the other as a control and tell me how each works out."

"I was given a dime a week from the time I was three years old. Of course, I had household chores, and I wouldn't get the full amount if I goofed off. My parents moved this up about a nickel a year; as an adolescent I was getting about five dollars a month for movies and extras. I supplemented this with lunch money by going hungry. I learned to make do."

"I'm impressed with your family's consistency. It may have been that your family was comfortable with this method. If you're comfortable with an allowance, try it for a while. In our family, we never had the right change. We just passed it out when they asked for something—if we thought it was worthwhile. My wife gave our daughters a clothing allowance in adolescence, made them shop around, and tried to bite her tongue when they made an obvious mistake. They really learned this way. We also learned that teenagers dress for their peer group, and there is little we parents can do."

"Well, I want to do it right."

"I don't believe there is a right or wrong way. Your whole family attitude is more of a determinant than the method. We put small change in a drawer in the kitchen. It is usually empty when I put coins into it; someone is removing that money for his own use, but no one in our house is a thief."

New Wives' Tale: If you nit-pick about money, your child may think it's more important than people.

"Begin your child in Sunday school early so he learns to believe in God."

"My twelve-year-old refuses to go to Sunday school. He's been going since he was four years old, and he always seemed to enjoy it. He loved the Bible stories and seemed to have a good concept of our religion, but something has turned him off. He hates to dress up. I think he's going with the wrong crowd at school and they tease him."

"And I suppose the more you push, the more he rebels."

"Exactly. Sundays are a battle. Our day of rest is D-Day."

"Do you go with him?"

"Not to Sunday school. We go to church, and he has his class during our adult service. Then we go home together. Sometimes we go to Grandmother's after the service for a brunch. We try to make the day interesting."

"I suppose it's getting boring for him. Maybe you could ask the minister if he could be rewarded for his long attendance by being an altar boy or carry the cross or sing in the choir or arrange the flowers or pour coffee. You somehow have to make him feel wanted, or that he belongs. Our minister revived our interest by getting us to read some of the service in the school. We felt important. We took turns passing the collection plate. Some of us got to teach a few of the little ones some Bible stories."

"Why can't he just follow the family example?"

"He's telling you he is growing up. Give him some options. If it seems to be a chore, he'll just hate it more and turn off religion entirely. Have you asked him why he doesn't want to go?"

"He says all the people in church are a bunch of hypocrites; they don't practice during the week what they promise they will do on Sunday."

"Maybe you can get him to do some good work during the week and not insist on his attendance on Sunday. He'll come back to it some day."

New Wives' Tale: Sunday school can only reinforce whatever Golden Rules are being practiced at home.

"Start training early; it teaches good habits."

I can remember my piano teacher telling me to thank my parents for the opportunity she was providing. I looked at her quizzically and thought, "Well, you crazy old bag!" But the idea might be worth playing with, and Mom had a good sense of humor.

"Mom, I want to thank you for the piano lessons."

Long pause.

"You'd better get cleaned up for dinner."

I was about five years into these lessons at age twelve and not once had I indicated that I was doing anything more than filial duty. This apparent change of heart was a new twist and overtly suggested that I was enjoying it. Mother knew I hated the piano; it was a boring drag to me. So this change made my mother suspicious that I was covering up some sneaky plot. She checked with the teacher, but all she got was the standard. "Oh, yes, he has much talent; if we could just motivate him to practice. . . ."

It was no surprise to my parents, then, that I was unable to play in a piano recital because I had "hurt" my fingers that very day. As a result of this, my intuitive teacher initiated a change of direction. Instead of the standard Chopin waltzes and Rachmaninoff's C# minor Prelude, my teacher suggested pianologues—poetry set to simple chords and connecting runs. The music was easy to master and I found I could replace the poetry with off-color limericks. It gave me a status in the neighborhood, helped my self-esteem, and even encouraged me to practice the piano more. My nervous system was okay; I just needed motivation.

Adolescents who are poor readers can be motivated with comics and "The Catcher in the Rye" much more satisfactorily than by forcing "Silas Marner" on them.

We have a daughter who is a little maladroit, or maybe better to say, loosely strung. We had heard, or believed, that the best therapy for this was ballet lessons. Maybe it was too much all at once, or maybe she sensed it was not her thing, but after the first lesson she tore into the house, threw the leotard on the floor, and announced, "Well, that's the end of ballet." A few four-letter words added weight to her decision, which seemed so final we let it stand. Today she is a fine potter.

I long cherished the image I got from a *Reader's Digest* article about the Alberghetti family—how they achieved a family solidarity because they all played musical instruments together. What a neat way to add purpose to a family! All of our family took lessons, but my singleness of purpose, optimistic encouragement, and cheerful but relentless drive netted two who play occasionally, two who could but won't, two who loathe the idea but listen, and one wife who says of the whole disaster, "I told you so." I justify my efforts now by saying at least they have an appreciation of what it takes to be a musician.

A mother calls: "I've signed him up for Little League and now he won't go. He seemed so enthusiastic at first but now just disappears when practice time comes. I can't let him get away with this or all his life he will think he can quit when things seem a little tough."

Another mother complains: "He's five years old and I've decided he should learn to swim. He put one toe in the water and began to cry. Each time we go he sits in the corner with his thumb in his mouth refusing to move. The instructors are pleasant and cheerful; they have bribed and cajoled, but nothing works. When they try force, he really fights. We can hardly get him to take a bath now."

One more: "My twelve-year-old sits around the house complaining that there is nothing to do, so I signed him up for a basketball clinic at the local athletic club. He says he goes but neighbors see him lurking around the park until it's time to come home. I'm furious with him, but I know he will just become more stubborn about anything I suggest."

I remember reading about 400 people over 95 years of age. A variety of life styles was represented, but the only common thing that seemed to keep these people going was that they all wanted to get up in the morning and go to work.

How do we motivate people, especially our children, to do something, anything? Dressing, eating nicely, cleaning the room, going to school, studying hard, reading, and having nice manners all seem to be so difficult to establish as firm habit patterns in children.

Somehow a child, or an adult, must believe that what he is doing or about to do is *fun.* Fun means that there is some built-in reward—money, a pat on the head, candy, or just a feeling of winning for a change instead of losing. My peer group was big on sports, and in order to be accepted I tried them all. I am left-eyed, right-handed, and generally klutzy, never quite playing up to standards. I even went out for football in high school thinking positive thoughts of self-mastery. I was about fourth team; that's the team the varsity squad runs its practice through. I remember "Truck" Halverson, a tackle, saying, "Smitty, we're coming right through you!" They did. (The coach said, as nicely as only coaches can, "Smith, you're not worth a fart in a whirlwind.") I rapidly developed some psychosomatic complaints and turned in my suit. I did get my letter, though; I was the cheerleader. I *had* to win somehow.

Behavior therapy is based on the premise that everything we do is learned. We learn better if we are rewarded for appropriate responses than if we are punished for unacceptable responses. What we don't know is the most auspicious time to get a child involved in some activity where there is a reasonable chance of success, so we, as parents, can reward the success. After age six or seven the child is usually so anxious for peer acceptance that he initiates his own activities. His motivation is group acceptance.

Office visit: "My husband was a success at everything: four-year letterman in all sports in high school and college, four-point grade average, student body president. He's well put together physically and intellectually. He seems disappointed in our son John, now nine years old. The boy is smart but built more like me. I've watched from the kitchen window with my heart in my throat as my husband pitched really fast balls at him which he often missed—perhaps because his eyes were filled with tears. Now John spends even more time in his room with his rock and stamp collections. All his playmates are younger than he; his only friend his age is another nonathletic type who plays chess with him."

The answer seems obvious. Why doesn't the jerk get off his son's back?

When a boy I am examining can leap up on the table gracefully, has a slow pulse rate (usually means he gets a lot of exercise), has straight legs (knees and ankles just touch when standing), and is thin and/or muscular, I ask about sports. Usually he is on the first team, is the fastest runner in the class (or second), or at least does well in sports and enjoys participating. If he is thin or fat and knock-kneed, somewhat maladroit, with pronated ankles, I ask about school or hobbies. He *may* do well in sports but it is unusual. We are, to a certain extent, trapped by our own bodies.

Later office visit with different mother: "We stopped Roy's music lessons after a year of screaming about practice. We let him drop out of Scouts because he said he hated it. He has a camera and takes beautiful pictures. He's always in the darkroom. He is pale and squints up his eyes when he is faced with anything more than a 25-watt bulb, but he's happy and his grades have even gone up. He's stopped smoking pot and laughs and has friends."

New Wives' Tale: Learning waits on motivation which waits on maturation.

11

"Sex Education Should Be Taught in Schools"

"My boy is a year old, and when I change his diapers he grabs his privates. His father is a dirty old man, but how could he have influenced him this early? Is the sex drive inherited? I slap his hands, shake my head and say, 'No, no, bad boy. Dirty!' But he persists. I have to change him occasionally; what can I do?"

This common worry is still a concern to mothers (more than fathers). It is difficult for me to believe the caller is not joking. So I give the old standard, "He is growing and exploring his body as well as his environment. His penis is part of his body, but is endowed with many more sensory nerves, just as his mouth, nose, eyes, and anus are. When he fools with himself, he finds it pleasurable and so continues the practice. If you make a big thing of his manipulation, he will be further encouraged because of the attention gained. He may have been drawn to it because he can now see over his fat stomach, and/or the opening itches because of some allergen or irritant in his diet, such as milk, orange juice, or chocolate. How about catsup?"

I'll say anything to distract the parents from some prejudice that genital manipulation is supposed to be sinful. They will punish him less if they think it is only an allergy.

It is true that many unwanted, rejected children find comfort in genital play; their bodies are more fun than people—so is sucking or rocking or hair-pulling.

"My daughter is four years old and she sleeps with a pillow between her legs. When I take it away she uses the blankets or rubs herself on the edge of the mattress. She gets a funny, faraway look in her eyes and sometimes falls off the bed. How do I teach her self-control so she won't be pregnant at age ten?"

Freud was right; children are "polymorphous perverse"—by our adult standards. "She has found an exciting part of her body at an age when this is considered normal and standard," I say. "You may be telling her by your taboo that this is a terribly exciting and adult matter, and so she will continue it. However, she may sense that she is bad for enjoying it; guilt about sex may return later to distort her marital happiness. Don't worry about her clutching her bottom at school; the other children will embarrass her out of it."

Children need to fool with *some* part of their bodies. They usually search about until they find an area that is pleasurable to diddle; part of the decision to remain at that place is determined by parental response. If a parent makes enough noise about thumb-sucking or nose-picking, the child may never get to bottom-clutching.

"My boys, aged five and seven, frequently disappear down the street with other boys and girls. I discreetly followed them one day. They have a clubhouse in an old garage. It is *not* group therapy. They are playing doctor, or house, or Playboy Club all kind of mixed up together. I know they are supposed to be curious about sex and body functions, but how much is too much? Where do I draw the line?"

"Maybe it *is* group therapy," I say, a little jealous. I vaguely remember watching a girl neighbor sit down to urinate. I don't remember any "good" emotion associated; it was something one had to do. You had to look. You had to find out if they were all the same. What if your parents found out? Even the threat of parental anger could not keep us from this curiosity; one simply *had* to look.

When our children were going through this age and the neighbors were calling to say something "awful" was going on in their garages, my wife, Julie, marched the kids all into the study, opened an anatomy book, and showed them pictures of a female bottom and a male bottom. "It's the same all over the world, so you don't have to keep looking." I'm sure they continued looking, but the neighbors didn't notice; the children had gone underground or had learned to be more discreet.

Julie and I may have suppressed the Peeping-Tomism too much, as none of our children want to go into medicine, the dream of curious children who play doctor. (One son, however, is an excellent photographer.)

We have two daughters, about a year apart. When they were small we happened to read in the paper an account of one of those dreadful situations where a six-year-old girl was lured away, raped, and killed. We were motivated to do something. I tried the following: "Now, you girls are standing here on the sidewalk going to school. I'm a stranger driving by. You don't know me. I ask you into the car and promise you candy; but you don't accept candy or rides from strangers. Okay?"

I drove up to them, swung open the door, and invited them in with, "Hello, girls. Come on in. I have some goodies for you." Instead of the anticipated negative response, I got, "Hey, it's Daddy!" They jumped in. "Where's the candy? Where are we going?" I drove them home. All I could do was give the old lecture about candy wrecking the teeth. We decided that luck may be an important child-rearing ingredient.

A wildly hysterical mother calls at 11:00 P.M. "We just got home from a movie and found our eight-year-old daughter crying in bed and the fifteen-year-old boy we use as a sitter looking sheepish. He must be guilty of something; he won't look us in the eye. I think he's done something to her, but we can't get anything out of either of them. Will you come over or do we call the police?"

These situations are tough; the most difficult thing for the doctor to do is to keep his cool. Examination of the child's genitalia may be more traumatic than the original episode. I talk to the girl privately and try to get her confidence; we are old friends, so it's easy. She complains of some discomfort in the area so I figure I must look. Things are calmer now. She allows me to look, probably because she has had yearly checkups including bottom inspections. All is okay. Now to get everybody to simmer down.

I was surprised to learn recently that about one-third of all children, boys and girls, have been molested, fooled with, diddled, or in some way approached sexually by an adult—girls usually by an exhibitionist and boys by a homosexual. In follow-up studies almost none of these children have had any problem with later psychosexual development, unless the parents and/or police have overreacted.

Armed with all these happy statistics, I can be very comforting in this incident, to the parents especially. The girl can't figure out what the big deal is. She was reared in an atmosphere of mutual trust, so she complies if an adult asks her to do something.

Fortunately there will be no charges filed and hence no court scene necessitating repeated questioning. The family of the boy has promised to get some help for him. (Good luck!) So the dust settles. A touchy spot for everyone to be in. I understand this problem never comes up in countries where there is a less restrictive atmosphere about sex.

I am also concerned that this girl might have somehow initiated this episode; I don't think she is truly neglected but I have a feeling she does not get all the affection she needs. The home is a little cold. She is just *too* charming with strangers. I think I detect a seductiveness here in the office during a routine examination.

Old Wives' Tale: "If a child says dirty words, you should wash his mouth out with soap."

"My son is cursing and swearing around here like a lumberjack. I don't understand. He used to be sweet and innocent. My husband and I let go with a good one occasionally—like when I burn my finger on the oven—but it just isn't our life style."

"How old is he?"

"Just six. He's so young to be so foul-mouthed. We've spanked him and even washed his mouth out with soap, but it didn't seem to help. He stopped for a while here, but the teacher says he's been bugging her with some goodies at school. It's very embarrassing. How do we stop it?"

"Well, the frontal attack didn't work. Tell me, is he doing well in school? Does he like it?"

"It's okay. He's a little overly active and would do better if he sat still and finished his work. I guess he needs this extra attention."

"I think you've hit on the reason and maybe the treatment. Are you strong enough to pay no attention to the dirty words?"

"I have to stop it, don't I?"

"Yes, but like so much undesirable behavior, it can be extinguished by ignoring it."

"No fooling! How can I ignore those awful words?"

"I have to convince you it will work, and you have to have something to do when he says 'bad' words. Get a piece of paper and write 'Naughty Words' at the top. Then every time he says one, you go make a check mark for that date. In a couple of weeks you will find the frequency rate will be cut from forty or fifty a day down to an acceptable five or six per day. Because it's an attention-getting maneuver, you must pay some attention to him when he's doing some socially acceptable activity. Read to him, have him cook with you, walk with him around the block looking for bugs. Do something fun with him."

"I'll try, but I'm getting to dislike being with him."

"Give it a couple of weeks. If it doesn't help, let me try. It's got to be fun. Get the teacher to do the same."

New Wives' Tale: If there is no audience, the actors won't perform.

"You have to solve an argument I'm having with my husband. He claims we do not have to build on to the house to give the children separate rooms. (Boy, eight;

girl, six.) I claim it is vitally important and he is just lazy. He could easily do it; he's a good carpenter."

I get the feeling that I am supposed to say, "Get them in separate rooms." Because our children grow up and live in our culture, they might as well be comfortable with privacy and modesty. The implication here is that the body is shameful and that sex is dirty or bad. This is unfortunate because it produces adults who are guilty and ashamed of normal sexual drives. Until our culture is able to feel a little freer about sexual feelings, we have to live with some of these attitudes. Fifty years ago you would have separated them in infancy; fifty years hence maybe parents will let them stay together until adolescence. In our society right now most parents cannot handle the normal sexual curiosity of children without anxiety or fear or at least overreacting. I guess my answer is, "Get them separate rooms." The advantage of a separate room is the provision of a haven for retreat. There should be some place where a child—or adult—can withdraw. A room, or at least an area of a room, should be provided that is the sole responsibility of each child in the family. How's that for a simple answer?

As the mother is hanging up the phone, I can hear her calling into the den, "He says you *have* to build another room on or we'll have incest on our hands!"

I guess what I was trying to say is that we are comfortable with our own sexual hangups only because we are used to them; it doesn't mean they are right for rearing the next generation. Keeping sex "guilty" is just another indication that we are unable to treat it as a natural human function.

Nobody ever calls to ask about the supposed harm to a child if he witnesses the primal scene. Maybe it never happens in a middle-class practice, but I suspect the parents are too embarrassed to ask about it. It seems obvious that it is occurring all over the world, apparently traumatizing only those children who interpret it as an aggressive attack. The viewer may identify with "aggressor" or "victim" and suffer some psychosexual thwarting, as he cannot cope with the anxiety engendered.

For those parents who have been "caught" by their children and were unable to consult someone, your explanation is supposed to go something like this: "You know how you kids get to roughhousing and playing wildly every once in a while. Well, your father and I love each other so much that we get to wrestling and rolling about and having fun. We're playing with each other, not fighting." If you act guilty, your child will think there was something nasty and hostile going on.

Remember, your child who has seen you having intercourse is saying to himself, "And they get mad at me for sucking my thumb!" So don't bug your child about his small pleasures. If parents can demonstrate kindness and affection toward one another, the child gets the right message.

Most of us are more comfortable with privacy, but these taboos about sexual behavior make it difficult for children to grow up with an accurate knowledge of their own genitals.

"My fully mature sixteen-year-old son has a girl friend that he is wild about. He's over at her house all the time, he glumps around our house, refuses to do anything I ask, and barely gets his school work done. Under these circumstances it is impossible for me to barge in on him and ask if he is taking the proper precautions, or if he needs to, or if he is in any kind of trouble. If I show *any* interest, he assumes I'm meddling. If I ask a question, I'm a nit-picker. I love him and trust him—I think—but things do happen. Should I pray?"

"If you are going to pray to prevent pregnancy, you'll be speaking to the wrong person. God is love. Boy-and-girl love is frequently followed by a pregnancy, which is exactly what God wants, if I understand Him properly. He wants the race to go on, and there is no other way. If you don't want them to get into trouble, you have to be the one to organize interruptions."

I hope it's changed, but a few years back a small town in the Midwest had the highest out-of-wedlock birthrate of any city in the state. The town elders knew that sex led to illegitimacy, so they allowed no moving picture theaters, bowling alleys, or malt shops. They even closed the drugstore at 7:00 P.M. instead of 8:00 P.M. because young people were gathering there. The assumption was that the young people would get up in the morning, do some chores, eat breakfast, go to school, come home, do some chores, eat supper, practice the piano, do their homework, and go to bed. Well, young (and old) people get together despite (or because of) obstacles, and if there is little else to fill the time they will have at each other.

The pregnant girls would go to the large University Hospital in Center City, have the baby, and then give it up for adoption. One girl was on her third at age sixteen. She was obviously a little bit responsible for what was happening, but you can fight off boredom and hormones just so long.

Keep them busy, but provide for some built-in control or interruption. Most do not ask for but really want some type of limit to aid their flimsy self-control forces.

It can't be too strict or too lenient and must mesh with the school and community code and curfew.

Until recently I didn't realize how subtly, but effectively, my parents provided supervision *in absentia* for my brother and me.

Son: (age sixteen and a half): "Mom, I need the car tomorrow night. There's this school dance I have to go to."

Mom: "What time does the dance end?"

Son: "Why do you have to know that?"

Mom: "Because. What times does it stop?"

Son: "Midnight."

Mom: "Okay. If you clean that Chinese whatnot in the hall, you may have the car. Be sure to check with your father. You must be home by one o'clock."

Son: "One o'clock! Aw, Mom, everyone else stays out till one-thirty or two."

Mom: "One o'clock. Your father has a reputation in this town. If something awful happens, it could mean the poorhouse."

Son: "Cripes!"

Because I had been programmed all my life for mutual trust, I got home at 1:03 A.M., a little tumescent but still "safe." Somehow Mother knew that we would all dance the last dance, we would go to the washroom, wash the grease off our faces, comb our hair, rank each others' dates, lay a few bets as to who would score, and try to decide where to go for the hamburger and malt. We usually ended up at some quickie place at the other end of town. By the time we were served and out it would be 12:40, just enough time to get the girl home and race home ourselves.

Mom knew that allowing one hour for driving and eating would preclude any heavy involvement at an age when sexual impulses might be poorly controlled or at least not dealt with properly or comfortably. It may be old-fashioned now, but in 1937 in our community it was appropriate.

When I complained that one hour was not enough time to eat and get the girl home without driving too fast, she suggested, "Why don't you stop at an all-night drugstore, and. . . ."

"And what, Mom?"

"And get a couple of Hershey Bars. You could eat and drive and save some time."

"Come on, Mom! Hershey Bars? She'd never go out with me again. Nor would anybody else."

"Just a suggestion."

It was not until a few years ago that I figured out that she was again helping me get through a bad age. She knew how hot and sweaty are the adolescent's hands. Who would grab and squeeze a girl with melted chocolate running down his wrists?

New Wives' Tale: Sex education is frequently taught in schools, but it is **learned** ***at home.***

"Little girls play with dolls; little boys play soldiers."

"My three-year-old girl doesn't like dolls or cooking or any of the domestic activities that girls are supposed to. We keep getting dolls for her, but she puts them in the laundry hamper or throws them under her bed. She likes to roughhouse, hates to dress up in a pretty skirt, and imitates trucks and airplane engines. Is she a freak or something?"

"I get the message that you're worried that she might become a lesbian."

"Well, it had crossed my mind. Where would she learn to be so masculine?"

"The final answer hasn't come to us yet about the

relative importance of heredity or environment on psychosexual development. We think some inherited tend encies are enforced by environmental influences."

"You mean we *made* her a tomboy?"

"Now, wait a minute. If I remember correctly, she's a vigorous, active, well-coordinated girl who loves to run and use her muscles. Call it exuberance. You naturally reward her curiosity, gregariousness, and adroitness. You throw a ball and she catches it. You say, 'good girl.' She loves the attention so she practices running, catching and action. She seems athletically adroit."

"She really is good at anything physical."

"That's the point. It's physical, not sexual. Our generation is crippled by the prejudice that muscular prowess is equivalent to sexual prowess."

"Doesn't that force her to be a hairy wrestler or size forty powerful Katrinka?"

"Not really. Being a ballerina takes incredible stamina. We do try to steer our children away from oddball pursuits so they won't become embarrassed. But I suppose a freaky child is an embarrassment only to his parents."

"What are we supposed to do?"

"Enjoy, love, encourage. You really have to accept her and her life style; then she will like herself. When her female hormones make her a woman, she will accept herself as a woman."

New Wives' Tale: God may be a female, so don't put women down.

"Pornography leads to sex crimes."

"What am I supposed to do when I find *Playboy* magazine in my twelve-year-old boy's room?"

"What *did* you do?"

"Well, I threw it in the garbage can and covered it up. What was I supposed to do?"

"Do you think he wanted you to find it?"

"Oh, I see! You think he's playing a game with me."

"Possibly. He probably knows you don't approve. He may be testing your limit. Maybe he feels guilty and wants you to punish him. Do you believe it will harm him?"

"Sure. Won't it? Don't sex criminals read this stuff and then go rape someone?"

"Someone got a grant to study this. Convicted sex criminals actually read *less* pornography than many other criminals or 'normal' citizens. You might even look on your son's interest as a normal, lusty, masculine curiosity."

"He appears to be turning out as horny as his father."

"I can't condemn him too much. After all, his pediatrician has a few interests in the same direction. Your job is to teach him a certain amount of direction. Maybe his curiosity can be re-aimed into photography, or dermatology or gynecology."

New Wives' Tale: Dirty-minded boys grow up to be fathers; if they had respect for their mothers, they will respect their wives.

"All sex offenders are dangerous."

"The neighbors and I believe that there is a Peeping Tom in the area. We're all frightened because most of us have children and are worried for their safety. When do they get aggressive and hurt people?"

"When an 'odd' person establishes his mode of acting, he rarely changes unless threatened or hurt. I would think you should be discreet but not necessarily overly seclusive."

"Shouldn't we set a trap and catch him somehow so he can be locked up and treated?"

"You might check with the police or the district attorney as to your rights or what protection the authorities might offer, but treatment is so difficult with these people that it is considered almost hopeless. Voyeurs, exhibitionists, and child molesters are supposed to be fixed at some early stage of psychosexual development; he is acting out his sexual age. A few are dangerous psychotics; I would hope you could find out whether this one is."

"Don't they castrate them in some countries?"

"Yes, but it is no cure. It's not the hormones from the testicles that drive them to do their thing; it's the odd ideas in their brains that are responsible for the actions. I understand that there are few Peeping Toms and exhibitionists in countries where there is more openness and nudity in the homes."

New Wives' Tale: Most sex offenders are the result of a constricting, unloving childhood; they can communicate only in an immature way. They want intimacy; the sexual pleasures are secondary.

"If a boy has sex with an adult homosexual, he will become a homosexual."

"I know it's late but I've just got to talk to you now. I'm just sick. My husband and I were out tonight and we came home sooner than usual. I don't know how to say this. Well, we hired a babysitter, a seventeen-year-old boy we know in the neighborhood. He is a nice, quiet young man—or so we thought. He didn't hear us come in. We didn't find him in the living room so I went upstairs to our son's room and caught him zipping up his pants and smoothing out the covers of the bed. My husband is furious and I'm just worried sick."

"What do you think happened?"

"I just know it was something disgusting. What should we do?"

"Is your son still awake?"

"No, he's fast asleep."

"And the young man?"

"My husband chased him out."

"We can worry about this problem later. I'm sure you'll be unable to sleep tonight, but I must find out from you your own feelings and beliefs."

"I've heard that if an older male excites a boy sexually, then the boy will become a homosexual."

"There has been a tremendous amount of research about this, and there is not one shred of evidence that this has been the persuasive event in the development of a homosexual."

"Really? Oh, I'm so relieved. But I feel so guilty that I left my boy with that freak."

"Don't be so hard on him. He does have a problem; he has acted immaturely and he needs some psychological help. But how will you handle your own son?"

"I'll just try to forget the whole thing and hope that he does."

"If your own sexual hangups prevent you from letting your son talk about the experience, then I must do it for you. Don't lecture. Try to set aside a quiet time tomorrow after school and get him to talk about it. Don't moralize. Don't condemn. Don't use the words 'right' or 'wrong.' See if you can detect some emotion in his speech or gesture. He must be allowed to work out any fear, guilt, or anxiety in the security of your acceptance."

"I can't accept what they must have been doing. I've got to let him know it was wrong."

"You don't even know what happened. Maybe you're assuming something. You've got to let him talk. Then ask, 'What do you think about it?' Give it a try. I'll back you up. Call me after your talk and let me hear what you've found out."

New Wives' Tale: A confused child needs a secure adult.

"If I don't have sex with my boyfriend, I will lose him."

"You've known me and my daughter since her birthday sixteen years ago and you often make sense. Help me with her adolescence."

"She's pregnant?"

"Ye gods! Not yet! Don't lay that on me. I'm calling before it happens or to prevent it from happening."

"She's covered with acne?"

"I wish she were and maybe they'd avoid her. No, she's an attractive, bright, warm, and friendly girl. We have always been open and honest with each other. We discuss things naturally and she usually lets me know if she has a problem. Her current boyfriend is a nice boy but he looks like he's after just one thing. After her last date with him she wanted to talk. She said he wants to go all the way with her. She likes him a lot and doesn't want to lose him—yet. She has friends who go all the way, and some lost their boyfriends and now feel very guilty or feel they are cheap whores. Other friends refuse to do more than neck a little and they have lost their boyfriends because they don't go farther. Can I advise her some way?"

"What did you say to her the other night?"

"I told her that her father and I are against it because it would cheapen her and might lead to VD or pregnancy. That's standard, isn't it?"

"Yes. Young people are living in a different society from the one we had, so our advice is usually considered old-fashioned, but *she* is the one that takes all the risks. You might give her some options, or at least some answers to his entreaties. The boy usually has a need to score, to achieve, so he can let his male friends know he is capable or can perform. He *may* also love her. When he says, 'If you love me, you'll do it,' she might be able to respond with, 'Love is not a matter of making demands.' If he cannot respect a refusal, it suggests what he thinks of her."

"What if he says, 'It's a natural thing to do'?"

"She could say, 'Is it love or lust? Is shooting someone an answer to anger?' "

"Then he says, 'Be a sport.' "

"Then she says, 'It's not a sporting arrangement if I take all the risks.' One expert suggested that a girl whip out a paper stating that he accept all responsibility and insist that he sign it. That might be as effective as pouring her iced cola drink in his groin."

"That would also end her dating career."

"There are so many factors involved here. I think the most important thing is that you two trust each other. No matter what happens you must be the accepting mother. If she decides to be sexually active, however, you must provide her with some contraceptive advice or equipment or pills. To become a mother at that age is a cruel reward to her, the baby, and society."

"I'm not sure I can hold *her* together through this when I can hardly hold myself together."

"It was ever thus: most boys are for it, most parents

are against it. The girl has to choose and live with her choice. Tell her she doesn't have to have sex with anyone if she doesn't want to."

New Wives' Tale: If you have sex with your boyfriend, you may lose him and a few other things.

"Acne will clear up after marriage."

"My son has a terrible case of acne at age eighteen. When does it go away? We've done all the diet changes, face scrubbing and lotion bit, but it continues. Can he get some hormone or anti-hormone shots to help? Grandmother says not to worry as it will clear up after marriage. He thinks he looks so awful that no girl will ever marry him."

"Acne usually goes away after age eighteen to twenty, but it is only a coincidence if marriage takes place simultaneously. A superstition relates acne with unreleased heterosexual activity. I remember leafing through an 1890 home health manual, and the only colored pictures were of a boy's clear complexion when he didn't 'abuse' himself compared with his pimply complexion when he did. What a lot of nonsense! Most adolescents have acne and most of them masturbate, but one does not lead to the other."

"Which am I supposed to worry about?"

"Let me call in some degreasing lotion and some tetracycline for the acne and let him take care of the other problem—if he thinks there is one."

New Wives' Tale: Acne can usually be controlled with medicine.

12

"When You Grow Up, You'll Thank Me"

Old Wives' Tale: "There are no bad children, only bad parents."

"We've spanked him, we've ignored him, we've bribed him, we've loved him, but we have no control. He runs the house. What do we do now? Can we divorce a child?"

Parents with clenched teeth confront me every day. They were once happy-go-lucky, fun-loving people who were anxious to experience the adventure of rearing a human being. They tolerated the pain, discomfort, worry, and sleepless nights because they were doing something for someone. But after a while the rewards don't quite compensate for the tiredness, headaches, and depression which demand daily aspirin and tranquilizers. The attitude of the relatives isn't very supportive: "Our grandchild would be better behaved if you weren't so nervous." These well-meaning people forget that the parents were relaxed and tolerant until this child came along to challenge their equanimity.

"One day when he was only four and a half months old I went into his room to get him for lunch and discovered the crib was empty! I panicked, thinking he had been kidnapped, but was relieved to find him on top of a chest of drawers. He must have pulled himself up on the crib sides, jiggled the crib over to the chest, and climbed up on top. Four and a half months! He laughed at my concerned face. My happiness at his safety was suddenly replaced with depression when I realized I had one of *those.*"

This description of a child's early life is not unusual to hear, but as doctors our ability to help is limited to such platitudes as, "He's all boy," "He'll outgrow it," "You've got to discipline him more," and "Good luck." We were not taught what to do; we were only told that this wild impulsive behavior is the direct result of ineffective imposition of self-control by the parents. These children have no obvious neurological impairment—they may walk and talk earlier than the average. They are frequently treated for worms, because they act as if there is something stimulating them, making them restless and wakeful. Something seems to be goosing them. Their formulas are changed frequently because they suffer from colic, or at least they seem to react inordinately to normal amounts of gas. Cuddling them seems to excite them rather than relax them; they cannot be rocked to sleep. They are exquisitely ticklish; horseplay with father becomes a frightening, painful experience.

At ten months of age: "I can't feed him; he insists on finger feeding, and it's a mess. I slap his hands but we just get to screaming and crying and the dog gets the lunch."

At fifteen months: "I can't say anything to him without triggering a tantrum. He falls on the floor, kicks his feet, pounds his fists, and screams like a banshee. Where did he learn this? We don't do this when we don't get our way. I throw water on him, I spank him, but it makes him madder. I go into another room to ignore him, but he follows me and has another tantrum. We're afraid to go out for an evening. He gets so upset we're afraid he'll have a fit for the sitter."

At two years: "Something has to be done. He has been sutured three times this last year. The police found him at 6:00 A.M. this morning over at the shopping center. I scolded him but I'm sure he doesn't know that he did anything wrong. His main words are 'no' and 'don't'; I suppose that's because they're the ones he hears most often. He won't toilet train, he won't behave, he won't nap, he won't go to bed, he won't do anything I ask. I think I'm reasonable in my requests and show my love for him many times a day. I need a little indication from him that I am his mother."

How can a parent discipline a child about running out in the street two hours after it happens?

If behavior therapy suggests ignoring bad behavior and praising good behavior, what do you do if the bad behavior is dangerous to health and there seems to be no good behavior to reward? If a parent rewards a pleasant smile does it matter that the child was smiling because he just hit his baby sister?

"I remember what you told me about trying to ignore unacceptable behavior, but twice this week I caught my two-year-old just in time climbing out the second-floor window. I grabbed his foot and hauled him back in. He now tries to get out the top of the window; I guess the bottom is no longer a challenge. Because I save his life, am I rewarding him by paying attention to him?

"After an episode of tumultuous behavior he throws

his arms around me and says, 'I love you, Mommy; I won't do it again.' Ten minutes later he *does* do it again and we repeat the sequence. It's as if an epileptic were apologizing for having a seizure or a diabetic were sorry because his blood sugar went up. Is it really that hard for him to learn self-control?"

Apparently it *is* for some children. Each age is heralded by a specific behavior pattern that may unbalance the most stable family:

10 months: separation cry

12 months: messy self-feeding

15 months: temper tantrum

18 months: "No"

2 years: whining, "Mine," "Gimme"

2 to 3 years: noncompliance in toilet training

3 to 4 years: use of dirty words

4 to 5 years: lying, cheating, stealing

Most children sail through these developmental levels with a minimum of struggle; they try the age-appropriate response, discover little reward for its use, and hence abandon it and move on to the next level, like a game of Stump the Experts.

"If a child shoplifts, he should be put in a juvenile detention home."

The following frequently repeated telephone encounter is an example of parental over-reacting to a normal developmental level.

"I was never so embarrassed in all my life. The local store manager called and said that they were holding my son Charlie until I got there. He wanted to talk to me about Charlie's shoplifting. Stealing, I call it. My husband will beat the stuffing out of him, and he'll be grounded for a year."

"Wait a minute!" How old is Charlie?"

"Five. But he's old enough to know better. We go to church; he knows the Golden Rule. What's gotten into him?"

"I can appreciate your concern. I assume if a parent reacts this way, she is normal. I would like you to cool off a little and try to understand the reason he probably did it."

"Why should he want anything? He's spoiled because we give him everything. That's the trouble!"

"Now, wait a minute. Human behavior is rather more complex than that. 'Taking things' at this age is so common that we usually assume it's a normal phase of development. He's learning to use his conscience and he needs to know how far he can go. He was caught, so he is supposed to file that bit of information in his brain. He tested the limits of his environment as he would test gravity. He found it. Now he should respect it."

"Don't tell me all kids do this."

"No, the hyperactive, blue-eyed blonds are more likely to do it. See something; pick it up. To them it may not be a conscious or premeditated activity, just a simple reflex, like a knee jerk."

"What do we do?"

"You and the store manager are the key people here. Arrange an appointment for today or tomorrow—you, Charlie, and the manager. Most managers have been through this so many times, they're fed up. They mainly want you to act as if you will do something. You must be concerned but not hostile. Charlie is supposed to look a little guilty and/or contrite. Some punishment —immediate and quick—is applied. Try: 'Charlie, you did something wrong. How do you think you should be punished?' A couple of days of no favorite TV programs might do. Then you have to *forget;* never bring it up again. He has to get the message that his behavior is bad; not that Charlie is bad. Too much attention directed to this might somehow reward him for doing it. At the same time you must reward him for some socially acceptable behavior."

"How do I keep my husband from killing him?"

"If you can't do it, get him to call me. Sometimes a man will take it from me when he can't from his wife."

"Okay, but I'm really nervous."

"Look on it as you did when he had a temper tantrum at eighteen months. If the problem is chronic, it suggests he thinks he's a loser or he has a bad self-image. This is usually the motivation when the eleven- to fifteen-year-old is shoplifting. That youth is waving a flag, trying to get someone to do something about his depressing 'I'm no good, so I'll do bad things' attitude."

New Wives' Tale: If a child shoplifts, it may mean he doesn't know where right stops and wrong starts and he wants to have the concept defined.

Psychologists dealing with disturbed families need a base line of pretreatment antisocial actions as a level with which to compare post-treatment results. Armed with clipboard, counting chamber, and graph paper, the parents add up the daily total of unwanted responses, say, of temper tantrums. It may be no surprise to learn that after two weeks of counting the wild floor poundings, the daily total may have been cut in half. Data gathering becomes the treatment. Since the parent has to turn around and make a check mark on the graph paper and click the counter, the child finds he is performing in an empty room without an audience. He figures, "What's the point?" and searches for another form of communication. Would an actor stop performing if no one came to the theater?

My wife, a reasonably normal woman, discovered each of the children could get her to react if they experimented with certain words: "nervous," "stupid," "fat," and "old." She knew she was not stupid, fat, or old, so she refused to react, but "nervous" got to her, and the resulting lecture with appropriate gestures and expressions was enough of a reward to encourage each child to repeat this frequently from age three until they and she became bored and it was defused. Dirty words were harder to ignore because some of the older neighbors really flipped when they heard any mention of the excretory organs.

Deconditioning works if the child is normal and the parents are convinced they can do it. Easily attainable goals are set. A pediatrician, psychologist, or psychiatric social worker must act as the rooting section.

Some children, maybe 20 percent, find they have struck a responsive chord in their parents and think: "Aha! This is it! I've got their number!" This is a mutual problem of a somewhat negative, noncompliant child with parents who may be depressed and discouraged with their own lives. They cannot afford to share a little of the love and trust they carefully hold for themselves. They may hate their child because he is the obstruction to their own fulfillment. These parents will lash out at any obvious, overt behavior that reminds them of their entrapment.

Sometimes it is the child who overreacts to his environment and sometimes it is the parents who overreact to the child's pushy behavior. If the parents are reasonably content with their lives and the child is "normal," behavior modification or at least acceptance of the child's developmental levels will allow child-rearing to be a joyful, rewarding phenomenon.

But what if the child is not normal? What is normal? What makes a child abnormal? A wealth of evidence now makes it clear that many children—maybe 20 percent—have a structural or chemical defect that does not allow the brain to function properly. Their intelligence is in the normal range but impulse control is insufficient. A child with a minor form might be a goof-off or underachiever. A severe form would be manifested by restless behavior and rapid-fire speech like that of many night-club and TV entertainers. Thomas Edison and Winston Churchill were like this as children. It is a relative, highly subjective phenomenon.

The following are some clues that the child may have this hyperactive trait or minimal cerebral dysfunction. Some obvious cases have all these irritating quirks to an exquisite degree. There are minor forms of the problem; the child may only be busy and ticklish. He may have no trouble in school until the seventh grade when he can't cope with extra homework. Stress from the environment always makes them worse or more noticeable so it appears that the environment is wholly responsible. They are better in a one-to-one human relationship. The environmental pressure will force a latent proclivity to become overtly disruptive.

Created much intrauterine activity

Has colic, is unresponsive to formula changes

Is a light sleeper

Overreacts to household noises, screams when the vacuum cleaner is on

Cries because he is crying

Cries himself to sleep every night

Sits, stands, and walks early; often doesn't crawl

Overreacts to frustration

Is difficult to cuddle

Seems on a different time schedule than the rest of the family

Temper tantrums go on "forever"

Feels better if nibbling; unable to eat a big meal

Is restless—constantly wiggling feet, rocking, squirming, bouncing, twitching

Talks compulsively and is usually shouting

Needs to touch and feel people and things

Is exquisitely ticklish

Has inordinate fear of doctor and/or possible pain

Cannot be reassured

Is accident prone; ignores gravity

Lights fires, "takes things"

Runs away, wanders off, forgets to return

Is easily sidetracked

These are physiological or chemical phenomena. They may be enhanced by environmental factors but they are not initiated by psychological forces. The defect that relates all these observed phenomena is an inability to disregard unimportant events, internal or external. It is as if every stimulus that enters the nervous system must be acted upon, like a reflex. They must touch all they see, discover the source of every sound, respond to a full stomach as if it were appendicitis. The doctor is surely a Dr. Frankenstein. A tickling game is a Chinese torture.

Some of these children may have inherited the tendency; they have little of the specific enzyme that produces the chemical that allows the impulse control center to function adequately. We know heredity is involved because the boys outnumber girls about eight to one. These boys are usually blue-eyed blonds and their fathers are more likely to be blue-eyed blonds who could not settle down in school. It is also known that birth trauma, anoxia, and prematurity predispose to the condition. Even where the enzyme and the chemical may be adequate, these insults may hurt the area of the brain upon which the enzyme acts.

These children act as if their parents have reared them without limits; they seem spoiled. Although a variety of psychological problems is present in families with these children, the amount of discipline imposed or limits set are usually much more than average. The children are frequently the targets of parental rage and they become battered. Physical punishment and/or verbal abuse produce anger or tremendous guilt.

"I'm no good," is a common remark of these children. The parents' usual response is, "We love you, but you could try harder." The child who thought he was doing his best develops a poor self-image and virtually abandons himself to his capricious nervous system. Truancy, stealing, delinquency soon follow in an almost predictable pattern.

Psychotherapy has been shown to be of little value; in many cases the behavior may worsen. Guilt may be erroneously laid on the parents. Behavior therapy with rewards to encourage positive social responses and impulse control may be unsatisfactory because it is difficult to find something to reward. Also, to be successful the reward has to be given almost simultaneously with the act.

Drug therapy for these children is the cornerstone of control—not cure or treatment—only control, just as a diabetic or an epileptic is controlled rather than cured. It allows the parents to deal with the child in a more normal fashion.

These children *have* a conscience but the neurochemical defect prevents them from using it. Medicine does not dope them: it allows them to use the part of the nervous system that mediates self-control. With the child's impulses under control, the adults in his environment can more freely and easily show some love and warmth and *acceptance.* Constant commands and questions like, "Where are you now?" "What are you doing?" "Come here to me!" "Go to bed!" "Eat your food!" "Stop wiggling!" "It doesn't hurt that much!" can be replaced with, "Hey! That's great!" "You're a nice boy!" "I love what the teacher said about you!"

The preservation of the precious self-image is the key to child-rearing. If the child gets the concept filed away in his temporal lobe that he is wanted and loved, then he has a better chance of becoming a reasonable, non-neurotic adult. He will always be restless and impulsive but he will be able to laugh at himself as he takes his place in the world. He may become an entertainer, actor, salesman, or even a pediatrician; he usually does better in jobs involving people, speech, and action.

If child-rearing is not fun, something is wrong. If everything the child does is an aggravation, something is amiss with the child or parents or both. Imitation is the best way for a child to learn self-control. If the reward system is not working and physical punishment is becoming a way of life, the child may be one of *those.* Blows make him angry; "putdown" words make him hate himself; violence at home leads to violence in the street.

New Wives' Tale: Bad behavior may be chemical.

"A healthy family should play together, stay together, and always see eye to eye."

"My fourteen-year-old son failed to make the team and got an incomplete in chemistry this term. The day both these things happened he came home seething with anger but his eyes were filled with tears. He was mad at himself for being a disappointment to himself. 'Why was I born?' he asked, slamming his books down.

"I realized he was depressed and life seemed pointless. Mine didn't seem much brighter, but I tried: 'Because we wanted you and loved you.' I know that is true, but the real truth of his origin was a planning error. How could I say, 'Your father and I couldn't sleep one night, and here you are!' That really would have sunk his waning self-image."

I assume this mother was telling me, the boy's doctor, because she wanted some reassurance that her fourteen years of mothering were not to blame. I pumped life into her so she could pump life into him: "Yeah, good, that's great, that's the way it is."

"Will he *ever* be ready to go out into the world? He seems immature about so many things. I can't protect and coddle him all his life."

On the other hand, the ones who seem to need more growing-up time are the very ones who leave early: "My daughter Joyce has run away. What should I do?"

"When?" I ask, trying to remember who Joyce is.

"Last night we had our usual argument about school, responsibility, and grades. I admit we did a little screaming, and she finally said, 'Shove it!' and walked out."

Now I remember who Joyce is; how could I forget? I have talked to her mother over the phone and in the office every month or two for the last thirteen years. Colic, night wakefulness, food refusal, breath-holding spells, accident proneness, wandering out into the street, disappearing at family outings, stubbornness, noncompliance, always complaining, have kept her mother tense and on the defensive. Her former pediatrician didn't help much; he vacillated in advice from, "You've got to get tough" to "Try ignoring her behavior; maybe it will go away." I'm surprised this family stayed with me so long; I suppose they figured I had at least kept her alive.

Joyce has a brother and a sister who, by contrast, are angels. They eat, sleep, have friends, and laugh more than they cry. They are, however, turning away from the family because it isn't any fun. "Oh, good, we're going to the beach; does Joyce have to go?" Joyce gets the easiest chores to do about the house but complains that she does the most. "Is she paranoid? She's been saying, 'Shove it!' 'Go to hell!' and 'Up yours!' since she was two years old."

About one in five children is built like this and destroys the dreams of his parents who knew there would be hassles but assumed that love would conquer all.

"She does some awful thing, so I discipline her. She responds with, 'You don't love me.' My response is a headache and/or crying myself to sleep. Is Flip Wilson right? 'The devil made her do it?' "

"Okay," I say, getting back to the immediate problem of Joyce's running away. "Did you call the police?"

"No, I thought that would make her even more hostile. I was hoping she would return when she got hungry and tired."

"That's a point, but somehow calling the police indicates you care enough to worry. Way down deep, Joyce is supposed to get the message that you want her home safe and sound. Of course, the police will indicate to you that you are an unfit parent and have not exercised enough control or have not taught her responsible behavior, but you've got to call. If they find her and you have not reported her as missing, they will really assume you're not adequate. Report her, get her back, and let me do a little counseling with her. I'm supposed to act as a kind, understanding friend who can accept her life style and build her self-image. We might try medicine to modify her impulsive behavior, but she'll probably think she is being poisoned and refuse it. If we can settle for an armed truce until she is older and maybe more mature, then at age eighteen you might want to open the door a little. Is there a relative with whom she might live who has a few of her traits?"

A girl like Joyce might have done better in the extended family of the old days; she could have related to a "funny" grandmother or to "different" Uncle Herman better than to her own parents. Her behavior might also have been less obvious if diluted in a larger household.

Parents generally are able to intuit their adolescents' needs for independence and allow and even encourage some freedom of thought and action. A few mistakes are educational.

"My daughter, aged fourteen, now a freshman in high school, refuses to wear the clothes I have bought for her. If I do manage to get them on her, she refuses to go to school, or if she leaves the house I'm sure she skips school. What now? I want her to look nice, and my taste in clothes isn't all *that* bad."

I respond, trying not to put the mother down: "Adolescents dress for their peer group. They want to be independent by conforming to new trends. Don't give in too easily. Give her something to complain to her friends about: Make her tuck her wrinkled work shirt in her blue jeans before she leaves the house, knowing she will pull it out when she's out of sight. Insist on clean underwear, though. How about a clothing allowance? Give her some motivation. Tell her she will get $25 a month for everything, and if she wants to buy a winter coat she'll have to save up for it. Check with the school, though, about a dress code. Most schools nowadays tolerate anything short of breasts or pubic hair showing. We have to have a few rules."

This sort of balance between autonomy and overcontrol may not work for children like Joyce, who sense that any rule is an occasion for direct and hostile confrontation. They overreact. But some parents overreact, too, and assume any surly mouthings of the narcissistic adolescent are a challenge to their caretaking.

They ground the experimenter for months; this only teaches the youth to be sneaky.

The "normal" adolescent in the "normal" household tries a few maneuvers to find the most effective way to disturb equanimity. It is not as if he attempts some aggravating ploy on purpose; some action or deed is "rewarded" by attention. However, the development of a negative ambience or feeling in the house is essential to the loosening of infant and childhood ties. It is subliminal but palpable.

I found my mother responded best to a form of passive aggression (perhaps based on a Scot background of silent stubbornness in the face of British pressure). Each Saturday morning my brother and I had an hour's worth of work to do about the house. My usual chore was dusting an intricate Chinese étagère. To do it completely required dental floss and Q-Tips. If mother said, "Just once over lightly," I did an exquisite job requiring two hours. If she said, "We're having guests tonight; do a good job," I spent ten minutes doing it once over lightly.

At age twenty I found it easy to go away to college to get away from the nit-picking.

How about the mother who says the last thing before her son leaves for a date: "Have a good time; do you have clean underwear on? What if you're in an accident and they have to cut your clothes off?"

We have a son safely into his sophomore year of college; getting him there was a five-year saga of mother-son interaction.

When he was thirteen years old and preoccupied with gaining the acceptance of his peer group, he once inadvertently left the bath towel on the floor after his usual 67-gallon shower. Apparently gaining points with his mother was secondary. After a dozen years of home maintenance lessons from a Scandinavian I would have thought that hanging up a towel would have been as automatic as breathing, but her response was immediate and appropriate.

"Who do you think picks up things around here? The fairies and elves? It's your *mother!*"

"Mom, I was going to pick it up."

I was drawn into this with, "Go talk to *your* son." I did.

He said, "Dad, I was going to pick it up." And I believed him. I reported to his mother that everything was straightened out. At least for 23 hours. A recurrence triggered a similar scene. I'm sure his mother felt that if she did not make a few household chores automatic, she would hear from a future daughter-in-law that somehow the upbringing had been deficient. Over the years they saw eye to eye on the war, politics, education, work ethic, and the like, but towel-picking-up could not be controlled.

Finally, at eighteen and a half, two weeks before college, he used up the last of the hot water and let the towel go again. It was too much. Another scene. He stood his ground. "Look, Mom, I got a 3.5 in high school, I keep my hair clean (albeit long), I don't smoke much pot, I only have two beers a week, and you haven't heard from any of my girl friends' parents."

"Yeah, okay," she considered all this thoughtfully. "What's the point?"

"Which one of these do you want me to change and I'll pick up the towel?"

"No deals! Get your clothes, your records, your skis, your bike! You're going to college."

She drove him down with teeth clenched the entire

thousand miles. He was dumped at the dorm. "Give me a call someday."

"See ya."

After two weeks of hot water but a feeling that something was missing, the phone rang. It was Eric. Depression and loneliness made him almost inaudible. "I have this terrible cold," he sobbed hyponasally. "I have to have a twenty-page thesis in by tomorrow and somebody stole my bike!" Things couldn't have gotten any blacker for him. Recognizing the diagnosis, I tried to help him in a practical way.

"Gee, that's too bad. Why don't you take an antihistaminic for your cold, shuffle a few old high school themes together—they don't expect big things from a freshman—and I'll look into the insurance for your bike."

His mother, sensing this was not telephone advice for a patient, came around the corner from the living room. "Who are you talking to?"

"It's Eric. His life is ashes. He's down the tube."

"Oh, let me talk to my baby." She melted the phone with all the beautiful things she had said to him eighteen years before when he needed her to feed, clothe, and cuddle him. Her soothings awakened an old memory in his temporal lobe; someone cares. His "cold" cleared up, and the thesis and bike problems became less formidable. His immediate concern was to hold the earpiece tightly against his head so his roommate would not hear his mother treating him like some little kid.

"Okay, Mom. Thanks. Okay. I'll check with you later."

As she withdrew from the phone she couldn't help asking, "Who's picking up the towels?" She must have pictured a dozen moldy, soggy towels lying on the floor.

I tried to clap my hand over the mouthpiece before it was too late. "Are you okay?"

"Sure, Dad, it's okay. *I* pick up the towels. Who else?"

In a flash I figured out what I had been witness to for the last five years. He had somehow forced his mother to nit-pick enough to allow him to leave his comfortable lodgings (record player, free food, electric blanket, private back entrance, hot water, etc.). He knew he had to grow up and get out. If there had been no intramural discomfort, separation anxiety would have been so overwhelming he might still be here.

He came back for Christmas vacation and got a booster after another towel-drop.

"Is this some sort of motel? Are you sure school doesn't start until the sixth of January? I thought all classes began on the second."

"Okay, okay."

We fed him food and love, taught him about gravity, fires, and freeways, gave him an education, and exposed him to some culture and humor and the Ten Commandments. All that is training for living elsewhere; he has a few things to do for himself. We'll always love him and welcome him back but he doesn't belong to us. He belongs to himself and the world. God lent him to us while he was growing up.

New Wives' Tale: From the moment of conception, everything is aimed at getting the child out of the house.

Epilogue

Just one more thing! Let me tell you what modern medical care is working toward. We have found that much of medical knowledge can be fed into a computer in such a way that some exciting results can be realized:

1. Consistently accurate and rapid evaluation could be made over the phone, enabling the parent to make a presumptive diagnosis of a child's condition.

2. The machine could set a worry level on the disease and suggest to the parent either that the doctor should be contacted or that home measures should be applied.

3. The data could be informational, providing criteria for a call-back. Temporal guidelines would allow the parent to know how long to "put up" with a sick child before seeking medical help.

4. This service could cut the doctor's phone call time in half.

5. The machine could be available night and day and could be "taught" to say, cheerfully, "I'm glad you called."

Cheerful accuracy, without putting you down for calling with an inane question at 2:00 A.M. If the machine told you to call me, then I would know you needed me and I would be more enthusiastic in my response. It would prevent us doctors from making you feel guilty.

The New Wives' Tales will be Old Wives' Tales in the next generation.

Index